KICK-START THE NEW YOU

HEALTH AND WEIGHT LOSS TIPS FOR AMAZING RESULTS

INGRID **MACHER**

WHITAKER
HOUSE

Kick-Start the New You:
Your Guide to Losing Weight and Staying Healthy
Published originally in Spanish under the title:
Al Rescate de Tu Nuevo Yo

Ingrid Macher
GetHealthyGetHot.com
FatLossFiesta.com

ISBN: 978-1-62911-618-1
eBook ISBN: 978-1-62911-619-8
Printed in the United States of America
© 2016 by Ingrid Macher

Whitaker House
1030 Hunt Valley Circle
New Kensington, PA 15068
www.whitakerhouse.com

Library of Congress Cataloging-in-Publication Data
Names: Macher, Ingrid, 1973- author.
Title: Kick-start the new you : your guide to losing weight and staying healthy / Ingrid Macher.
Other titles: Al rescate de tu nuevo yo. English
Description: New Kensington, PA : Whitaker House, 2016.
Identifiers: LCCN 2015041453 | ISBN 9781629116181 (trade pbk. : alk. paper)
Subjects: LCSH: Reducing diets. | Weight loss. | Food habits. | Reducing diets—Recipes.
Classification: LCC RM222.2 .M1813 2016 | DDC 613.2/5—dc23 LC record available at http://lccn.loc.gov/2015041453

1 2 3 4 5 6 7 8 9 10 11 **W** 23 22 21 20 19 18 17 16

Dear God, this book is the result of the inspiration and strength You have given me throughout the years. I want to dedicate it to You, because it is thanks to the new opportunity You gave me that I was reborn to serve You and begin my mission of making the world a healthier and happier place.

Dear beautiful women of my life, I also want to dedicate this book to all of you! Through your messages and words of encouragement over social networks, emails, and YouTube, you continue to motivate me every day, and I am committed to holding your hand in this quest to rescue the gorgeous women who live inside each one of you. I want to tell you that while we remain united and concentrate our strength and faith, we'll never give up, and our conviction to be healthier and happier will triumph above all.

I love you and want you to remember that my strong arm is always there for you!

—*Ingrid Macher*

CONTENTS

ACKNOWLEDGMENTS

Jeff, your love has made me the woman that I am today. When I thought there was no hope of escaping the heavy and lonely life I was living, you showed up, my saving angel, my soul mate, my partner and husband who came to rescue me and Paula and teach us that there is a world of possibilities. There are no words to express the great blessing you have been in my life! I thank you for your immense love, your support, and your commitment to our family. You are the love of my life! Without you, none of this would be possible.

My two beautiful daughters, Paula and Mia: I want to thank you for every smile and for every word of encouragement, because you are my best cheerleaders. With your love, you always make my days so bright and make me stronger for the battlefield, ready to succeed.

To you, Dad, because thanks to your sacrifice and your hard work, you gave us a life full of happiness. Your teachings and your example have always been my model for honesty and humility. Thank you for being my inspiration.

To you, my beautiful mom: I thank you for your sacrifice; despite your physical limitations, you were always a brave woman. God has given us the most precious gift to heal our wounds and start a new life: forgiveness. I love you! Thanks for showing me that there is always a way to achieve what we want, if we are indeed determined.

Finally, I want to thank everyone who opened the doors of their homes, who spread my message through the media, and who have driven me to continue this mission of love and health. To all producers, journalists, photographers, and special friends who have joined me in this journey, and especially to you, Daniza Tobar, for trusting me and letting me be part of your book *SOS Mamá Soltera* and for helping me edit mine; thank you for your love and trust.

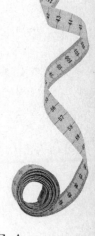

WAIT!

BEFORE YOU CONTINUE, I HAVE A SPECIAL GIFT FOR YOU!

I want to thank you and congratulate you for your willingness to take control of your health. I am sure this book will help you change your life, the same way it changed mine.

And as a thank you, I would like to give you this free e-book of slimming and revitalizing juice recipes for a healthier life.

Just visit: www.KickStartJuices.com

INTRODUCTION

Welcome to the new "you"! Congratulations on making the decision to change your life!

You have just taken the first and most important step to lose weight and be healthy. I am here to tell you that you *can* change your life! Making lifestyle changes may be intimidating, and may also seem impossible, but it's not! It is actually very easy. I know, because I did it.

My name is Ingrid Macher. I am the owner and founder of www.FatLossFiesta.com. I started this business as a hobby, but after seeing the happy, euphoric, amazed faces and even the tears of so many great people I helped through the years, I knew this is what I wanted to do for the rest of my life.

I am a holistic health coach and certified personal trainer, health motivator, mother of two beautiful girls, and your best ally. I have spent years learning what works and what doesn't work when you are trying to lose weight and recover your health.

And in this book, I am excited to share with you my secret of how I lost 50 pounds in 90 days, and how I have been able to keep them off throughout the years!

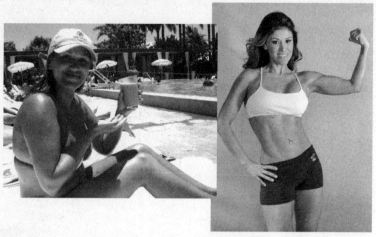

If you've ever wanted to lose weight, this is your chance and this book is your guide. I assure you that if you follow my advice step by step, you will achieve the results you desire.

My passion is to help people change their lives. Your life can be one of them.

Don't think of this as a diet regimen. Instead, use it as a manual to begin your new lifestyle. And remember, through this journey, you are not alone—we'll do it together!

So, are you ready for the new you?

OK, let's begin!

MY STORY

I was born in Bogotá, Colombia. I was raised with all the strictness of local traditions, including dietary traditions. I come from a family in which every woman had to, at some point, deal with weight issues, including obesity. So far, I am the only one that has been able to overcome those issues.

In 1992, at age 19, I decided to migrate to Puerto Rico; I've always wanted to live by the sea. Bogotá is a beautiful city, but it is cold, and I love the sun and the beach. Puerto Rico, *La Isla del Encanto*, or the "Island of Enchantment," was the ideal place for me. My sister lived there already, so it was a natural choice. I studied communications and graduated as a publicist from the Universidad del Sagrado Corazón; I got married for the first time and had my oldest daughter, Paula.

However, I was never able to work in my field; I wanted to continue studying, but then I got divorced and my plans changed drastically. With my daughter still very, very young, I decided to start a new life in Miami.

When you arrive in the United States, as a professional, you think life will be easier, but you soon discover the harsh reality! I quickly realized that I had to find a way just to survive. I worked really hard as a single mother for seven years; I had two full time jobs and worked seven days a week. My life was not easy.

But in 2004, my life changed completely. In the elevator of my apartment building, I met Jeff Macher, the love of my life. My soul mate! Within a month we were officially dating and three months later, he asked me to marry him. Up until then, one of my job requirements was to stay fit, tan, and very thin. However, my new marriage and a great economical time for us filled my life with such sweet moments—and many thoughtless moments of excesses.

We moved to Las Vegas to start a family. We were doing great! We bought a mansion and for many years, I lived the life that I never could before. I stopped working and visited the most exotic places in the world, eating and drinking. Not long after, I was pregnant with my second daughter and along with this new blessing came new challenges.

As my overweight condition and poor diet began to show its consequences, my health began to deteriorate. When I was six months pregnant, I developed asthma, a silent killer that affects millions of people around the world. The asthma attacks were constant, and my fairy tale began to disappear before my eyes. I vividly remember Christmas night, in the seventh month of my pregnancy, when asthma almost took my life. I was alone with my mother; my husband had gone to visit my in-laws. It was a tradition to spend Christmas together, but that year unfortunately, due to my health condition, I couldn't travel. God knew I had to stay at home.

At about 10:00 p.m., I began to cough nonstop. My breathing was shallow, and it was becoming difficult to talk. My poor mother, distraught, did everything she could. I honestly thought my life was coming to an end, but I wasn't discouraged. I asked God with great intensity to help me hold on until my husband returned. So I spent the night in anguish and suffering, but with the hope that everything would be fine the next day. Finally, dawn came and I was able to get in touch with Jeff. He could see the gravity of my condition, so he boarded the first plane he could and managed to get home in three hours. By that point, my face was starting to turn purple from the asthma attack. He took me to the emergency room right away, where I was revived.

I survived, and after nearly two months in bed and in treatment, my daughter was finally born, a blessing from God. However, I have to confess that despite this experience, I still didn't realize that I had to be healthier—and I didn't know how to do it, either.

And then, the economic downturn of 2008 hit.

Overnight, we woke up to a different financial reality. We had to start all over, and we decided to move back to Florida to begin again.

And that's when I noticed that my bad health had taken a toll on my body *visibly*. When my husband and I began to reunite with old friends whom we hadn't seen since our move to Vegas, their facial expressions said it all. They didn't mince words, either: "Wow, you've changed! You look chubbier." Those comments were a bitter surprise for me. Up until then, I had everything I needed in order to be happy, to the point where I forgot to take care of myself. It was then that I realized that I needed to change my life and be healthier.

The "South Florida" stigma of looking great welcomed me back, and it also gave me the motivation I needed to change my life. But it wasn't easy. No diet plan worked for me!

Finally, after trying out tons of different methods to lose weight without success, I decided to investigate and put together my own program, to fit my specific needs.

My first step was to create my means of motivation. I pulled out old photos of myself that were taken when I was thin and fit. Whenever I looked at them, they motivated me to be the happy and attractive woman I had always been. I also purchased a pair of jeans that were the size I was before getting married. I hung them on the closet door as a reminder that I once was that size—and I could go back to that size again. These tricks and many others helped me become the person I am today.

Then, I designed a plan of attack and executed it.

After three months of dedication and discipline, I reached my goal: I was the same confident and healthy woman I had always been. I not only recovered the figure I had when I was young, I was also able to control my asthma and never had to use medication again!

My lifestyle change motivated me so much that I decided to become a certified personal trainer and a holistic health coach. With all this new information, I started to encourage my closest friends, teaching them how to take control of their lives and be healthier. Soon, I discovered that this was my calling. My passion to motivate others was so big and contagious, that, without realizing it, I started to help complete strangers that, today, are also my friends.

I love what I do. I love being able to bring a positive message and educate others. With God's help, my goal is to teach people to lead a healthy life, to be more active, and above all, to truly understand that nothing is impossible to achieve. You can achieve any goal you set for yourself, if you have the right attitude.

Today, I have been fortunate enough to be described as one of the prominent experts in health, exercise, and nutrition; not only in the Spanish market, but now in the American market as well, as dozens of specialized American magazines use my advice in columns and articles.

Thousands and thousands of people consult with me every day from different countries through Twitter, Facebook, or my website. That's why I invite you also to be part of my family and join me in my mission of making the world a healthier and happier place.

You can find me on:

Facebook: http://facebook.com/Burn20

My blog: http://GetHealthyGetHot.com

Twitter: http://twitter.com/lose20

Instagram: http://instagram.com/lose20

Youtube: http://youtube.com/GetHealthyGetHot

My program that covers everything you need is at: http://FatLossFiesta.com/

Are you ready to change your life?

Let me help you regain your confidence! Follow me and you'll get daily tips and secrets on how you can take control of your life!

Nothing is impossible; I promise, you can do it! I'll be here to help you achieve all your goals. So...let's get started!

Chapter 1

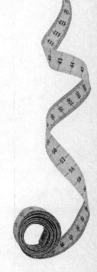

YOUR #1 ENEMY: NEGATIVITY

Today we are going to have a history class and go back in time. We are going to talk about what was going on with me before I was able to lose weight and find the "magic formula" to keep it off.

When I was overweight, I used to make the same mistake over and over again; a mistake that cost me tons of effort and kept me from progressing in my fight against those extra pounds. You are probably making the same mistake. So the information that I am about to give you can make your fat loss journey a whole lot easier and a whole lot more effective.

What was my mistake? The mistake that I kept making over and over was to *fill my head with negative thoughts.*

I allowed my desire to give up to take over my thoughts. My belly was a lot bigger than what I wanted it to be. But instead of concentrating on my diet and exercise regimen, I kept thinking of how unhappy I was. I let my mind fill up with all those negative thoughts.

I kept saying to myself, "I have a huge belly!" "I will never have the flat tummy I've always wanted!" and that was the sad truth. Because as long as I kept thinking this way, I would never be able to give my body the boost it needed to change.

If I only focused on my flabby belly, my mind could only hear those words, "flabby belly," and accepted that as reality.

I was basically telling my body to stay fat!

You see, before you take control of your body, you need to first take control of your mind.

The mind is a powerful thing. But you have to think of it as being a small child. You have to control everything it is exposed to. Would you allow a three-year-old child to stay up late watching horror movies? Of course not! All of those images would stay in his mind, scaring him and making it impossible for him to sleep.

You have to treat your subconscious the same way. If you expose it to all those negative thoughts, it will "get scared" and focus only on those thoughts. But if you give it something positive to focus on, your mind will join your body to help you achieve your goal.

There are two ways of doing this.

First: stop surrounding yourself with negative people.

If you are surrounded by people who complain all the time, especially about their bodies, you will, eventually, start complaining about your body, too!

If you have a friend who only tells you how much she hates her "bat wings," you are naturally going to start telling her about the things you don't like about your body. But this behavior is not effective; all you are doing is reinforcing the areas of your body you don't like. So, recognize the negative people in your life—and stay away from them!

Second: create a habit of changing your negative thoughts into positive thoughts.

Focus always on the positive side of things. If it's a rainy day, don't complain; think of it as an opportunity to stay in and watch a movie. If you feel you are "too fat," instead think about how you're going to lose that weight quickly.

As soon as you notice a negative thought, substitute it with a positive one. Once you make this a part of your daily routine, you'll be training your mind and your body to help get you that slender body you've always wanted!

This is the key to losing weight almost effortlessly.

MAKE YOUR MIND DO ALL THE HARD WORK FOR YOU!

When your mind and body are balanced, your training routines will become easier, the cravings disappear, and you will begin to burn fat without noticing it. We are the mere image of our thoughts. Our body doesn't have another choice than to follow what our mind does.

You don't believe me? Try this: next time you are in a bad mood, I want you to smile. This will probably be the last thing you want to do, and you may think it's silly, but it doesn't matter; I only want you to try. Force yourself, if necessary, but continue smiling and wait for the magic to happen. Believe me, it will happen!

It's all about the connection between your mind and your muscles. Our mind has been trained, during our entire life, to associate a smile with a good feeling. It doesn't know any different!

So, when you make yourself smile, no matter how you are feeling; your body doesn't have a choice but to produce the emotions that follow the smile. Our minds have been trained for it; you smile, and it assumes you are in a good mood, and works tirelessly toward that.

This is why, along with your weight-loss journey, you are going to start each and every day with a smile. Every day should be a celebration. You are alive and able to smile!

I know the huge difference this will make on your results. When I started my challenge of losing weight, I decided not to be like other people that allowed themselves to fail. I wasn't going to fake a positive state of mind, there was just simply no room for negativity—hidden or not!

UGLY THOUGHTS LEAD TO UGLY BODIES

It is a sad truth, but most people who decide to lose weight give up before they reach their goal. And honestly, most of them were probably not going to be successful. They were doomed from the beginning. Why?

Because they didn't face the challenge with the right mind-set. Instead of focusing on all the benefits they'd be *gaining*, they focused on everything they had to *give up*. They were angry when they couldn't eat their favorite foods that, after all, are the same foods that betrayed them over the years, the meals that have stolen their natural energy, and the ingredients that have filled them with toxic pounds.

When going to the gym to work out, they did it lazily, trying to finish the exercises quickly. Their minds were already giving up while their bodies were doing the exercises. But this is not going to happen to you. You really want this change; and to make that change a reality, you are already filling your mind with positive thoughts.

SPIRIT UP!

Keeping a positive attitude is crucial in order to succeed. You'd be surprised! In all my years of training both myself and others, I still don't get tired of saying that—and I still don't think I say it enough!

When you think big, big things will happen, they happen. But when you mentally *quit* or get discouraged, you'll start going backwards.

Sometimes the results you achieve are not the ones you wanted or hoped for. You may feel frustrated because you are not getting the results fast enough. All of these frustrations, all of these doubts may lead you to think negatively and may even get you to consider quitting this goal. After all, we are only human, and sometimes we get discouraged and lose faith in ourselves.

However, you have to understand that at the beginning of this journey, *any* result is a good result. Don't respond by *quitting* in your mind; instead, just remind yourself, *I'm still moving forward!*

TIPS TO KEEPING
A POSITIVE ATTITUDE

Motivational books have played a huge role in my weight-loss journey. I read all types of inspirational quotes and poems. Sometimes, you just have to pick up your mind out of what's bothering you and carry it toward something positive—sometimes, that's all that is needed to stand up again.

A trick I did at the beginning of my weight-loss journey was to take a picture of myself and put it on the refrigerator door. Then, I found an *old* photo of myself, from when I was younger and thinner, and put it in the bathroom mirror.

Every time I opened the refrigerator door to get some kind of unhealthy food, I had the brutal reminder right in front of me, reminding me *not* to eat that piece of chocolate cake.

Every morning, while I was getting ready to go to work, I would get dressed in front of the mirror and see how much closer I was to being as thin as I was in the picture. I was transforming into a new person. And believe me, it *felt* every bit as good as it *looked*.

Another one of my tricks was to keep the clothes I used to wear. Even though those clothes hadn't fit me in a really long time, I kept them to prove to myself that I could fit in them again. It really didn't matter if I wore them again or not, I just wanted to know that I *could* wear the same size again.

But all of these tricks are useless unless accompanied by positive thoughts. I am here to help you as much as I can, but I can't make you believe in yourself. If you don't believe it, you won't be able to find that inner strength.

But I know, since the moment you picked up this book, you already believe in yourself.

VISUALIZE

There are many ways of achieving things you never thought possible. Do you think I always knew I could have the body I have today? A little part of me really thought I could, but a huge part of me didn't think so at all!

But thanks to this "mind trick" I played on myself, I did it!

Get ready to discover my secret weapon. Of all the things I've shared with you until now, this is probably the most important:

Visualization.

It is incredibly powerful! Moreover, it is responsible for everything mankind has invented. Before creating something, before turning it into a reality, you have to visualize it. You have to know what you are trying to create.

But your vision must be clear. The clearer you visualize yourself and know exactly what you want to look like, the more real your chances will be of achieving it.

This book is all about your goals of becoming a better version of yourself. It's not about competing with anybody, for this shows a negative mind-set, and we know how dangerous that can be! If you are forty years old, it is not realistic for you to try to visualize yourself as a seventeen-year-old. We are not that young anymore, and you have to accept that! If you don't, it will lead to a pile of negativity.

But this doesn't mean you have to lower your standards. No matter how old you are, you are completely capable of developing an amazing body, with tons of energy and even toned abs to show off at the beach. All of this is possible; I am living proof of it!

I just want to make sure you have clear and realistic goals. I wouldn't want to take you down the wrong path.

SETTING REALISTIC GOALS

Now that we have that clear, let's talk about how you are going to visualize the *new you* and make it a reality.

First, we need to find a goal to inspire you, something clear and specific that you can imagine achieving. The more you see, the more you'll believe. And believing is everything.

For me, my goal was simple…I wanted to fit into one, specific, sexy, way-too-small pair of jeans.

As you probably already know, jeans were designed for fit women. They are made to button at the hip with no problem. Well, these specific jeans gave a whole new meaning to the so-called "low-cut." When I lived in Las Vegas, there were women everywhere wearing these jeans, and they definitely had the perfect bodies to go with them.

It was one of the most frustrating things I've experienced in my life. I wanted to wear those jeans so much! But no matter what size I tried, even the largest size out there, they just didn't fit. No matter how hard I pulled, they simply did not go past my thighs.

I, however, was not going to give up. I was determined to fit into those low-cut jeans and not die trying. I knew that if I could fit into them, I had achieved the body of my dreams.

I will say it again: if you can *visualize* your goals, you will be able to achieve them.

So I bought a pair of low-cut jeans and hung them in my closet as a reminder, and a constant motivator. I was *determined* to fit those jeans. Every so often, I would take them out and try them on, and every time they went up a little higher than before. I was a little bit closer to my goal.

After three months, I could pull them up completely and close the button.

They fit me!

There are no words to describe what I felt that day. It was just priceless! I literally cried. They were tears of joy, and they scared my wonderful husband—he saw me crying and didn't understand what was wrong with me! It was when he realized I was wearing my jeans that he understood they were tears of happiness. He gave me a hug and congratulated me because in three months I had dropped from a size 32 in normal pants to a size 26 in tight, low-cut jeans. And I was able to do it because I *visualized* it, and then I set a realistic goal.

You have to do the same! Find something that motivates you. It has nothing to do with brands. It has to do with your goals and what you have to do to achieve them.

Maybe it's a bathing suit, or a little black dress, or how about that tank top to show off your toned arms? It is your choice. But whatever it is, hang it in a place in your room where you can see it every day.

Allow yourself to see the future and see yourself looking amazing! With a clear picture of what you want, you'll always be reminded of your goals, and you will not be able to miss your workouts or break your diet as often.

Try on your motivator outfit to see your progress. You don't have to get obsessed. You don't have to try it every day—be reasonable with yourself. Maybe try it on every three or six weeks.

Of course it will not fit the first time, perhaps not even after several attempts. But as you progress, you will notice yourself moving closer to the goal.

Whenever those "jeans" come up a little more, you've reached a great achievement, something you should celebrate. Before you know it, they will fit you and you will look amazing! Being consistent never fails.

Chapter 2

NO MORE EXCUSES!

When we are not 100% convinced of something, then we haven't visualized it yet, and we certainly don't have a positive attitude about it. You see, there is always some excuse to prevent us from doing what we need to do in order to change our lives, especially when those changes are to improve our health.

But you have to understand that by making excuses in your head, *you're only cheating yourself.*

As soon as I stopped making excuses and decided to really educate myself on this healthy lifestyle, I adopted changes. For the first time, I saw results, and I saw that my body was slowly becoming the body I've always wanted.

The only way to get rid of the excuses is to be able to notice them flitting around in your head. I came up with a cheat sheet that will help you to identify the excuses you make. Here are some of the most common excuses that will sabotage the *new you*:

1. **I do not have time or energy for exercise.** It is important to remember that healthy eating and exercise increase your energy levels *incredibly*. This means that you will not only have energy to do all you have to do during the day, but you will also have leftover energy for other activities. If you're one of those people who have a hard time checking off your to-do list, you should start exercising. I promise; you will be able to do *more*, not less!

2. **I don't want to stop seeing my friends because I'm on a diet.** Friends always find a reason to go out and celebrate with dinner. You don't have to say no; instead, when dining out, simply choose one of the healthy menu options. Nowadays, most restaurants offer a healthy section on their menus, including baked, broiled, or grilled options that aren't full of flour. Resolve to choose a healthy option *before* you sit down, however, or you might find yourself tempted to order the greasiest item on the menu! More on that later!

3. **I don't want to stop eating my favorite foods.** I agree, it is very sad to think you'll never eat that rich chocolate cake that you like so much! But I have good news: a healthy diet is not as bad as you think. As it turns out, you do not have to leave these foods altogether! Eating them occasionally can actually help you burn more fat. Eating a healthy diet that includes whole foods throughout the week allows you to have a cheat meal once a week. In other words, *never say never*.

4. **I don't want to go to the gym because I'm embarrassed to exercise in front of others.** The truth is that when you're in the gym, nobody cares what you're doing! Everyone is so focused on doing their exercises to look and feel better; they don't even realize you're there. But

if you are too uncomfortable, you don't have to go. Just do some exercises at home. You can do fat-burning routines using your own weights; you can also do squats and lunges in all their variations for an excellent workout.

5. **Healthy foods are very expensive.** You don't have to be a millionaire to enjoy healthy meals. Think about it this way: junk food will have you looking for more to eat within an hour. However, if you eat lean protein and fiber-filled foods, although they are a bit more expensive, they will keep you full for longer and help you to eat less—and in that way, saving money!

When it comes to losing weight and leading a healthy life, we have to constantly be very careful about the decisions we make. Remember that every bad decision you make will delay you from achieving the ultimate goal. So, forget the excuses! I assure you that every day, it will become easier and easier to continue.

15 MYTHS ABOUT EXERCISE AND NUTRITION

I probably don't have to tell you how confusing it is to look for a weight-loss plan. In my first battles looking to lose weight and keeping it off, I found tons of information. Over and over, I'd read about the "new formula for the ideal weight" and there I was, buying it and following it step by step. And *nothing*.

Then I'd learn on television about miracle pills that make you lose weight without dieting or exercise, about magic belts that are instantly slimming, about exercise machines that are absolutely guaranteed to help you lose weight, or about some diet that has never ever failed. I would get my hands on any new method advertised to lose weight—but the result was always the same. A number on the scale that *wouldn't budge*.

Does this sound familiar?

We hear and read so much about nutrition and exercise! Some say to do one thing, others disagree; so who is telling the truth?

The truth is that we are all wonderfully different and some options work better on some bodies than others. But there are many essential healthy *lifestyle tips* that work well for all.

So let me go ahead and bust some of the myths that keep us from losing the weight we want to.

Myth #1: The fewer meals you have a day, the more weight you will lose.

Fact: When you don't feed your body with the nutrients it needs, your metabolism slows down. On the other hand, eating smaller portions several times a day keeps your metabolism running and accelerated to burn more calories when you are not eating. So, don't skip any meals!

Myth #2: You have to spend hours and hours at the gym every day.

Fact: It is not about how much time you spend exercising at the gym or at home; it is about the *quality* of the exercise. Search for routines that work as many group muscles as possible and that you can complete in about twenty minutes. That's it!

Myth #3: The fewer calories, the better your results.

Fact: Eating fewer calories only delays your weight-loss process because it slows down your metabolism. Stop counting calories and allow your metabolism to be activated by eating more throughout the day in smaller portions.

Myth #4: The number of hours I sleep does not affect my weight loss.

Fact: The less you sleep, the less you'll move the next day, and the fewer calories you'll burn. If you want to burn as many calories as possible during the day, make sure you sleep at least six to eight hours every night. Additionally, lack of sleep affects your levels of leptin and ghrelin—hormones that control your hunger. If you don't sleep enough, it can actually make you feel hungry!

Myth #5: Low-sugar foods and carbs like saccharin and other sweeteners help me to lose weight.

Fact: Studies have shown that any foods low in calories that contain sweeteners and saccharin are the most fattening, because they "allow" you to eat larger amounts and they increase your cravings for sweets.

Myth # 6: If one diet does not work, it makes sense to try another.

Fact: You will not lose weight if you keep jumping from diet to diet. You will only get more and more frustrated and create bad habits for your body with so many changes and without the adequate nutrition.

Myth #7: If you are a woman, exercising with weights will make you look manly.

Fact: This is only possible if you train with really heavy weights and spend a lot of time at the gym. You would also need to eat very large amounts of food so that your muscles grow like a man's. Exercising with hand weights will just create a sexy, toned, and very feminine body!

Myth #8: Exercise machines are more effective than free weights.

Fact: The truth is that exercise machines are designed for men, and it is a bit harder for us women to manipulate them. Free weights, however, give us the freedom and balance we need.

Myth #9: You don't need to exercise every day.

Fact: Even though you are not obligated to, it is better if you exercise every day. You will burn more fat, tone your muscles, and have more energy during the week.

Myth #10: If I sweat, it is because I am out of shape.

Fact: Sweating means you are an athletic person; it means your body is working at its maximum power and you are eliminating toxins.

Myth #11: Drinking water makes you fat.

Fact: Drinking water doesn't add calories. To the contrary, it helps control your appetite and expands your stomach, stimulating the feeling of satiety. Besides, if you don't drink water, you will become dehydrated and your body will not function properly, even slowing down your metabolism. You simply must drink at least eight glasses of water a day to keep your body working correctly, and if you drink ice cold water, you will burn even more calories.

Myth #12: Ab workouts are the best exercises to lose belly fat.

Fact: Abdominal exercises are not designed to eliminate fat; they are meant to tone your abs. Instead, do high intensity exercises that involve your abdominal muscles and other parts of your body. I assure you; you will have rock hard abs in no time.

Myth #13: Running is better than walking.

Fact: Running and walking are the same. The only thing that makes a difference is the speed at which you do it; they burn the same amount of calories.

Myth #14: Proteins make your muscles grow.

Fact: Protein shakes help your muscles *recover* after exercising; eating a lot of protein will not somehow magically grow your muscles.

Myth #15: Oily fish, avocados, and nuts should be avoided because they are all full of fat.

Fact: Yes, they are full of fat, but they are good fats; the kinds our body needs to help us fight the bad fat in our body.

FORGET THE SCALE!

I know people who come up to me all the time to tell me they are getting discouraged because they are not losing weight.

And my first question to them is: how do you know?

They look at me as if I am crazy and then respond, "Because I still weigh the same!"

I laugh at that answer, and always try to let them know how deceitful scales are! You will weigh more at night, after exercising and eating healthily, than in the morning. This doesn't mean that you gained weight. The scale is affected by what time you eat and by the amount of water your body retains. It even gets affected when we women get our "monthly visit."

Don't determine your success by the number on the scale. Pounds are not a very reliable indicator of whether we've slimmed down. Sounds weird, right? Keep reading and you'll know what I mean.

INCHES VERSUS POUNDS

The best way to know if you are losing weight or not is through your clothes.

If you feel your pants come up a little easier, you are on your way. If you can finally zip that little dress all the way up, good for you! This is how you should determine your success in your weight-loss journey. At the same time, if you feel your pants are fitting a bit tighter, then you know you must change something in your eating habits or exercise routine.

Even if you didn't lose any weight, but your clothes are fitting better or you are more flexible now, then you definitely lost some inches.

Lost inches are your best allies to keep you motivated every day!

Those lost inches that we begin noticing around the waist, hip, breasts, etc., are a more effective and stimulating marker than a scale. Another trick that really helped me throughout my process was to take pictures every three weeks in a bathing suit. And every time I saw results, I felt a lot more motivated and I kept pushing!

UP THOUGHTS OR DOWN THOUGHTS?

You also need to measure your success by your thoughts. That's right; you just need to pay attention to what you are *thinking*.

Maybe since you started this weight-loss journey, you have opted for taking the stairs at work. That is great! It was probably a little tough at the beginning, you may have reached the top out of breath, and your legs were killing you the next day. But this is normal if you want to get back in the game. And after a couple of weeks, you were able to go up the stairs easily. This is a small but significant victory that you need to take into account!

Remember to give yourself credit and consider those small victories your achievement. Don't be so hard on yourself. If you are, your confidence level may drop. And I know exactly how that feels. Once my attitude changed for the better, so did my body!

Chapter 3

YUMMY, YUMMY IN MY TUMMY

Laugh all you want, but I actually love food! I am one of those people who won't stop smiling after trying something delicious.

It is precisely because I love food so much, that I want to clear its bad name and reclaim its reputation: *Food is not your enemy!*

Food is not your enemy; food is amazing, fun, delicious, stimulating, diverse, and so much more! Food is the source and the essence of all the nutrients that our body needs for energy.

People who blame food for their weight gain should really blame themselves for choosing the wrong foods. Let's clear something up: not all foods are created equal. It all depends on what you eat, how you eat it, and when you eat it.

DIETS WILL NEVER GET YOU THE BODY OF YOUR DREAMS

I can only imagine your face when reading this title. But I am about to save you from an unnecessary frustration. If you have 10,

20, 30 or more pounds to lose, and you want to lose them once and for all, then it is important for you pay attention to what I am about to tell you, because the answer is not as obvious as you may think. If it was, you'd probably be at a healthy weight and wouldn't be reading this book. But the truth is that you continue to struggle with your weight.

Why? Because when it comes to losing weight and keeping it off, *diets don't work!*

I understand if you think this is crazy. It is the complete opposite to what you have been told: "if you want to lose weight, eat less and reduce the amount of calories you consume in one day."

This theory sounds pretty simple, right? But if you've ever been on that diet, then you know this theory never works.

You want to lose weight fast, so you reduce your caloric intake, and at the beginning, it works. You are taking your body to the limit to lose weight. And yes, you do lose some weight; it may not be the great transformation you had hoped for, but it's a start!

The problem is that your body is very smart, it adapts quickly, and it hates change. Your body cares more about keeping you alive than looking good in a bikini. Once it realizes it is getting less food and has less energy (which comes from the calories we eat), it'll start to save them by slowing down your metabolism.

So, when you consume fewer calories, you will also be burning fewer calories. This is where you get so frustrated. The scale stops "working," your clothes begin to fit a bit tighter, your progress comes to a halt and you have no idea how to begin again.

What can you do? You are practically killing yourself from hunger; therefore eating less is not an option. Since you are eating so little, you don't have the energy to exercise. You are trapped, there is no way out, and it is only a matter of time before you give up and go back to eating the same way you used to.

Study after study of scientific research has shown that, when people stop dieting, they gain all the lost weight back. How depressing, right? It gets even worse: if they didn't get the appropriate nutrition while they were dieting, their metabolism starts to suffer. And without a healthy, active metabolism, once they start eating the calories again, they gain back even more weight!

I have been in that vicious cycle more times than I'd like to remember. It is actually painful to think about how, if I had known back then what I know now, I would have saved myself from all that frustration.

There is a way to eliminate excess fat, without going hungry. You can achieve those rock hard abs without feeling deprived of your favorite foods. Believe it or not, you can have your dream body without any "diets." There is a way to lose weight while enjoying delicious and healthy foods to satisfy your hunger.

The day I discovered this, my life changed forever.

What's the secret? Learning that food is not your enemy, and learning how to eat, when to eat, and what to eat. Let's start with learning about the different food groups.

POWER UP WITH PROTEIN!

When it comes to losing fat, protein is one of your most powerful weapons.

It is an essential nutrient that your body uses to maintain every cell in your body. Other than water, protein comprises the largest part of your body by weight (around 16%). It is the building block that makes up our bones, blood, skin, muscle, cartilage, hair, and nails.

Protein is used to build and repair tissue, keeping us healthy and allowing us to recover from our workouts. It makes us stronger and helps us to build that lean, sexy, shapely muscle that makes us look amazing!

So how are we going to get it into our eating routine?

Proteins are made up of compounds called amino acids. There are twenty-two types of amino acids and your body needs all of them to function properly. These amino acids are broken up into two groups: essential and non-essential.

The eight essential amino acids cannot be produced by our bodies. They must be provided by the foods we eat. The fourteen non-essential amino acids can be made by our bodies, as long as we provide it with the right nutrients.

Both groups are important; so important in fact, that on your new eating plan you are going to include a protein-rich food in every meal you eat!

There are two types of protein: complete and incomplete. Complete means that it contains all eight of the essential amino acids. Incomplete proteins are missing one or more of these acids.

Most of the time, sources of complete proteins are going to come from animal products. Because of this, people often refer to them as "animal proteins." Sources of complete proteins include:

- Meat
- Fish
- Poultry
- Cheese
- Eggs

- Greek yogurt
- Chia seeds
- Seitan
- Tofu
- Protein powder

A lot of these sources also contain fat. When it comes to the animal proteins, I like to stick to the lean proteins, which include chicken, fish, turkey, yogurt, and eggs. But there are definitely times to include the fattier proteins such as red meat, as you do need some fat in your diet (which I'll explain in a later chapter).

Next up, we have the incomplete proteins. These are often referred to as the "plant proteins" since they mostly come from plants. Like I said earlier, these lack one or more of the essential amino acids, but it doesn't mean that they aren't important! Some of these protein sources include:

+ Beans
+ Chickpeas
+ Nuts
+ Peas
+ Lentils
+ Sunflower and pumpkin seeds
+ Green peas
+ Quinoa
+ Hemp seeds

As for combining them to form complete proteins, here are some combinations that I find work well:

+ Grains with legumes (almonds and chickpeas)
+ Grains with dairy (Greek yogurt and pistachios)
+ Legumes with seeds (lentils and pumpkin seeds)
+ Nuts with legumes (peanuts and chickpeas)
+ Dairy with seeds (Greek yogurt and sunflower seeds)

Once you decide which sources of protein you enjoy eating most, you're going to want to make sure you include a source at every meal. Proteins, in addition to helping build and repair our muscles, also help to blast fat by burning calories. This is because it takes your body a lot of energy to digest them. While they contain 4 calories per gram, your body will burn off 30% of these calories just during digestion!

And considering how filling most protein sources are, you don't need to eat a lot to feel full and satisfied. That's why it is so important to eat protein often; getting full on fewer calories allows us to drop the fat without ever feeling hungry. So make sure to get your protein in every meal.

DON'T CUT OUT THE CARBS SO FAST!

Next up we have carbohydrates; which, you'll learn, aren't the evil fat-causing villains that the media portrays them to be. .

When it comes to losing fat, there are always myths that spread like wildfire and become so widely known that most people believe them to be true. One of the most powerful is the myth that you should avoid carbohydrates in your diet at all costs. With all the hype that's been out there promoting low-carbs diets, it seems like just looking at a piece of bread is enough to make you fat.

Well, I'm here to tell you it's just not true! Eliminating carbs from your diet is an extreme measure that should never be a long-term plan. You see, carbs are one of the body's main sources of nutrients. Your body uses carbohydrates as its primary source of energy. When you digest carbs, your body breaks it down into glucose. This glucose is then used by your cells, tissues, and all of your organs, storing it in your liver and muscles until you need it.

So, you definitely need to have carbs in your diet. Without them, you won't have the energy you need to go about your day and enjoy your workouts.

But what most people don't know is that all carbs aren't created equal! Carbohydrates can be broken up into two groups: simple and complex. And in order to get the biggest benefits out of eating them, you need to eat the right type of carbs at the right time. Keep reading, I'll explain.

SIMPLE CARBS

Simple carbohydrates provide quick bursts of energy. They are made up of sugars called glucose that your body uses for energy. Unfortunately, they usually don't provide any of the other vital nutrients. A lot of simple carbs are found in foods that were processed and refined.

Simple carbs spike your blood sugar levels since they are digested so rapidly. This causes your body to release insulin in order to remove all the sugar being released into the bloodstream. This rapid release of insulin causes the sugar to be stored as fat.

Some examples of foods containing simple carbs are:

+ Fruit juice
+ Milk & milk products
+ Yogurt
+ Table sugar
+ Corn syrup

+ Candy
+ Cake
+ White flour (pasta, bread, baked goods)
+ Sodas
+ Most boxed cereals

To make it worse, many of these simple carbs are loaded down with added sugars. An effective way to avoid added sugars is to read the ingredients label of the foods you buy.

Look for these ingredients as added sugars:

+ Corn sweetener
+ Corn syrup
+ Brown sugar
+ Dextrose
+ Fructose
+ Fruit juice concentrates
+ Glucose
+ High fructose corn syrup

+ Inverted sugar
+ Lactose
+ Maltose
+ Malt syrup
+ Molasses
+ Sucrose
+ Sugar
+ Raw sugar

Other tips to avoid these types of sugar are:

+ Drink water instead of sugary sodas.
+ Drink only 4 oz. or ½ cup of 100% natural fruit juice, instead of an artificial fruit drink.

+ Opt for fresh fruit as dessert instead of a piece of cake—which often contains tons of added sugar.

+ Choose cereals without any added sugar or with less added sugar, such as oatmeal or all-bran cereals.

COMPLEX CARBS

Complex carbs include whole grain breads, vegetables, and legumes (beans and lentils). These sources provide more of a constant, sustained energy, allowing you to keep energy levels stable and your hunger satisfied for longer periods of time. They are also usually packed with more nutrients and minerals than simple carbs.

But this group of complex carbohydrates can be broken down even further. There are two different kinds of complex carbs: starchy and fibrous.

Starchy carbs

Starchy carbs, predictably, consist of starch, that is broken down by the body into simple sugars. Examples of these carbs include:

+ Brown rice

+ Sprouted grain bread (such as Ezekiel bread)

+ Oat bran bread

+ Rye bread

+ Potato and sweet potato

+ Whole wheat pasta

+ Peas like lentils and chickpeas

+ Beans and legumes

+ Whole grain oats

+ Whole barley

+ Oats

+ Muesli

+ Couscous

+ Bulgur (cracked wheat)

+ Whole grain cereal

+ Wheat bran

+ Buckwheat

+ Millet

+ Quinoa

+ Triticale

If you want to use starchy carbs for energy, you should eat them at breakfast and lunch to provide your body with the energy to get through the day. The negative of eating starchy carbs is that they're high in calories. You want to avoid them later on in the day so the extra sugar isn't stored as fat.

Fibrous carbs

Fibrous carbs will make up one of the most important parts of your eating routine. They are packed full of nutrients, while remaining low in calories, which means that you can eat a *lot* of them, eating until you're full (at any time of the day), without worrying about packing on any pounds.

Some examples of fibrous carbs include:

- Apple
- Celery
- Plum
- Apricot
- Cucumber
- Prune
- Artichoke
- Dill pickle
- Radish
- Asparagus
- Eggplant
- Spinach
- Broccoli
- Grapefruit
- Strawberry
- Brussels sprout
- Lettuce
- Turnip greens
- Cabbage
- Onion
- Watercress
- Carrot
- Yam
- Orange
- Cauliflower
- Pear
- Zucchini

As you can see, basically all fruits and veggies fall into the fibrous food category. The fibers these foods contain are crucial to keeping you healthy and lean. The fact that they are so low in calories means you can eat them in bulk to control your hunger.

But the benefits go beyond that. Fiber has been shown to lower blood cholesterol levels and prevent and improve constipation. It serves as your digestive system's special helper, sweeping up toxins and eliminating them from your body.

Now that we know this information, we're going to have fibrous vegetables in every meal we eat. Our bodies will thank us for it.

And since we're talking about fiber...

WHY DO I NEED FIBER?

Did you know that less than half of the population consume the proper amount of fiber? The ideal amount of fiber we should include in our daily diet is 20–35 grams. Most people receive less than 14–15 grams per day.

We get most of our fiber from foods such as fruits, vegetables, nuts, legumes, seeds, and grains. It has been shown that eating a high fiber diet helps reduce cholesterol levels in the blood, improves and prevents constipation, and slows the digestion process. Fiber reduces the rate at which foods pass through our digestive system, making it easier for our body to digest food.

According to Joanne Slavin PhD, obesity researcher at the University of Minnesota, large amounts of fiber can help to regulate blood glucose and insulin levels. This explains why people who take in more fiber tend to weigh less and are less prone to gain weight as they age. "The best protection is at the highest fiber intakes—at least 25 grams a day [is] recommended for women," says Slavin.[1]

---

1. Joanne Slavin, as quoted in Elaine Magee, "What You Should Know About Fiber," *Take Note*, Accurate Clinic, August 2009, http://accurateclinic.com/docs/Accurate-educ_Fiber.pdf.

Eating the right amount of fiber-rich foods can lead to a healthier lifestyle. This can help control your weight, reducing the risk of both colon cancer and type 2 diabetes. It can also slow down the buildup of cholesterol in the arteries, and it is one of the most effective remedies to protect our heart health.

Here are some examples of delicious, fiber-rich foods:

Bran (whole wheat, brown rice, oats): For breakfast, eat half a cup natural cooked oats. To add some flavor, without the extra calories of sugar, sprinkle a dash of cinnamon. Brown rice is always a great option for lunch, just before hitting the gym.

Flaxseed and sesame seeds: For a delicious snack, you can add some flaxseed to your fruit and yogurt.

Edamame: These vegetables are a fiber-rich snack, but be careful with the sodium content. Choose a low-sodium option and enjoy half a cup between lunch and dinner.

Dried tomatoes (dehydrated): Add flavor to your sandwiches, stews, or even chicken with these delicious vegetables, for some extra fiber.

Nuts (almonds, walnuts, pistachios, etc.): These nuts also contain healthy fats essential for a balanced diet. You can eat them with some fruit or yogurt to get the vitamins and nutrients you need in every bite.

Beans and grains: Add some black beans, green beans, white beans, or pinto beans to brown rice. You can even mix these with a little roasted garlic, bell peppers, dried tomatoes, and herbs for a healthy, fresh, and high-fiber salad.

Here is a list of foods high in fiber so that you can have a better idea:

Fruits

- Guava
- Apple
- Pear
- Raspberry
- Plum
- Orange
- Papaya
- Nectarine
- Banana
- Strawberry
- Kiwi
- Blueberry

- Cherry
- Grapefruit
- Mango
- Peach
- Mandarin orange
- Melon
- Watermelon
- Pineapple
- Raisin
- Grape
- Blackberry
- Honeydew melon

Vegetables

- Sweet potato
- Peas
- Brussels sprout
- Cooked corn
- Winter squash
- Artichokes
- Broccoli
- Carrot
- Asparagus
- Romaine lettuce
- Cauliflower

- Spinach
- Zucchini
- Cooked green bean
- Beet
- Bell pepper
- Lettuce
- Tomato
- Celery
- Onion

Grains

- Amaranth
- Black barley
- Tri-color pasta
- Barley
- Millet
- Quinoa
- Brown rice

- Black quinoa
- Couscous
- Whole wheat pasta
- Oats
- Whole wheat bread
- Sprouted grain bread

Legumes

- Beans
- Lentils
- Chickpeas

- Broad bean
- Edamame
- Tempeh

Nuts and Seeds

- Peanut
- Soy nuts
- Almonds
- Peanut butter
- Almond butter

- Pistachios
- Sunflower seeds
- Flaxseed
- Chia seeds
- Wheat germ

It is not always easy to include high-fiber sources in every meal. But if you include fiber-rich foods, you will gradually reach the daily recommended value of 30 grams a day. Your body will quickly adapt to the benefits of fiber and will thank you for it!

TRY THESE TIPS TO BOOST YOUR DAILY FIBER INTAKE.

- Eat whole fruits more often than you drink fruit juice.
- Include two veggies at dinner.

+ Keep a bowl of washed and ready-to-eat veggies in your fridge, such as carrots, cucumbers, and celery, for a quick snack.

  + Do one meal with legumes instead of meat.

  + Choose whole grain foods more often. A good guideline is to choose whole grains for at least half of your grain choices.

EATING FAT WILL NOT MAKE YOU FAT!

Now, we are going to talk about one of the most controversial subjects in nutrition. Another myth that has been tossed around is that eating fat makes you fat. Just like the myth about carbs, this one has been sabotaging people's weight-loss results for years. It's just not true!

What do you think our brains are made of? You may be surprised to hear that two thirds of your brain is made up of fat. And it needs a healthy intake of fat in order to function correctly.

Without the proper fats in our diet, it is hard to maintain a healthy positive mood. There have been some studies done that linked a low-fat diet to a higher risk of depression and even suicide.

A study published in the *British Journal of Nutrition* followed a group of dieters who switched to a low-fat diet. It found that making this switch brought them a 25% increase in depression and hostility!

Another study done at the University of Maryland Medical Center found that deficiencies in healthy fats can cause mood swings and depression. They also found that fats play a vital role in stimulating skin and hair growth, maintaining bone health, regulating metabolism, and maintaining the reproductive system.

Fats sound pretty important, don't they? Yet so many people are putting their health in jeopardy because of bad advice they read in a magazine. In case you haven't caught on, let me be clear: you need fat in your diet to be healthy!

YOU NEED FAT!

Fat provides us with energy and allows us to absorb and utilize vitamins. It helps improve our hair, skin and nails. It keeps our moods balanced and our brains functioning correctly.

But you need to know that all fats aren't created equal. While healthy fats bring us the amazing benefits we've been talking about, unhealthy fats can cause health problems.

There are two types of fats: saturated and unsaturated.

Saturated fats are generally unhealthy and can be found mostly in animal products and dairy. Saturated fat can be found in:

+ High-fat cuts of meat (beef, lamb, pork)
+ Chicken with the skin on
+ Whole-fat dairy products (milk and cream)
+ Butter
+ Cheese
+ Ice cream
+ Lard

Eating too much of these fats has been linked to high cholesterol, and that can lead to a heart attack. On your new eating plan, you're going to limit the amount of saturated fat you take in.

Instead, you're going eat *unsaturated* fat. That's what provides all of the benefits we talked about earlier. Most unsaturated fats come from fish and vegetable sources. They are essential to our health. Our bodies can't naturally produce them, so they must be provided through the foods we eat.

These healthy fats play a huge role in our weight-loss goals by keeping us healthy and functioning properly.

Examples of these healthy fats are:

+ Olive oil, grapeseed oil, sunflower oil, peanut oil, sesame oil, safflower oil, and avocado oil

+ Avocado

+ Nuts (almonds, peanuts, macadamia nuts, hazelnuts, pecans, cashews, walnuts)

+ Sunflower and sesame seeds

+ Flaxseed, chia seeds, hemp seeds

+ Fatty fish (salmon, tuna, mackerel, herring, trout, sardines)

+ Tofu

+ Pumpkin, zucchini, and other vegetables

Some people who can't get the fat they need regularly in whole foods will take fish oil in capsules and combine with exercise so the fat-burning enzymes work better. But if you like fish, instead of taking the supplements, you can eat salmon or tuna, which are both high in omega-3 fatty acids.

FOOD LABELS:
AN EXTREME CHALLENGE

Every so often, the Food and Drug Administration (FDA) and the Department of Agriculture (USDA) spend millions of dollars trying to design the best nutrition label for every food. What for? The idea is to provide consumers with the most complete information of the nutritional value of the products, so that everyone can make the best possible choice.

However, as the market has become more globalized, the borders have also opened for foods from around the world, and despite my opinion that imported foods should have similar labeling rules, the nutritional labels are only subject to the regulations of their country of origin. When you purchase a product, keep in mind that if it was imported, it may not contain all the nutritional information that you are used to.

When you read the label of the food you purchase, you can find a lot of important information. And although these labels seem easy to read, knowing how to interpret them may not be as simple as you thought.

WHAT SHOULD WE PAY ATTENTION TO?

First of all, before reading the label, look at the expiration date of the product. Is it still safe to eat? Also check how you're supposed to preserve it; does it require freezing, refrigerating, storing at room temperature, or storing in a dry place to avoid contamination? It is also important to look at the recommendations once opened. For example, canned foods generally need to be removed from the can, and if you have leftovers, you must store it in another container with a lid and refrigerate it.

Second, read the list of ingredients. Either you or a member of your family may suffer from allergies to certain foods. Many times, the problematic ingredient is not actually listed; however, the product has been processed in the same machinery or facility as the ingredient. This is a common difficulty for people allergic to peanuts or gluten, for example. If this is indicated on the label, don't buy the product.

Now, on the nutritional information label, pay special attention to:

Portion: The portion listed corresponds to the average amount a person consumes in a meal. The amount appears as a household measurement (cup, tablespoon) and next to it, in brackets, the amount is written in units of the metric system (grams = g, cubic centimeter = cc, etc.).

A common mistake is to grab a can of soup or a packet of crackers, glance at the label, notice that the levels of calories, sugar, fat, etc., aren't too bad, and then eat the whole thing without realizing that the product is comprised of two or even four servings! We've accidentally eaten twice or even four times what we intended to.

Calories: The amount of calories in a food product is roughly equal to the energy supply, which I will later discuss in detail. As a general rule, to measure calories more effectively, take into account the portion and calculate the energy value according to the calories that 100 grams of a product contributes. A helpful rule of thumb is that a food with more than 200 calories per 100 grams is quite high energy; a food with no more than 100 calories per 100 grams is relatively low energy.

Fats: As I've said a few times, it's not about trying to find low-fat products, but rather about paying attention to the types of fats. A food product of about 100 grams should not have more than 30% of trans fat (low-fat products should have no more than 10%). However, if the percentage is higher than 30% in saturated fat, trans fat, hydrogenated vegetable oil, or partially hydrogenated vegetable oil, it is better to leave that product on the supermarket shelf.

If we want to keep our cholesterol in check, we can look for products that contain monounsaturated and polyunsaturated fatty acids that, unlike the bad types of fats, are a source of great benefits.

Carbohydrates: Unfortunately, labels don't specify if the carbs are simple or complex; however, it's likely that the carbs on the label come from sugar. As a general rule, it is not recommended to eat foods that have more than 10% sugar per every 100 grams. For those who suffer from diabetes or high triglycerides, it is of course very important to check the ingredients for any sugar, fructose, sucrose, or even honey.

Note that 10 grams or more of sugar per 100 grams is considered high; 2 to 10 grams of sugar per 100 grams is moderate; and less than 2 grams of sugar per 100 grams is considered low.

Fiber: On average, adults should consume about 30 grams of fiber a day to keep our body functioning properly. Fiber not only contributes to the digestion of food, helping our intestines function properly, but it also determines the amount of glucose in our body and helps us to feel satisfied faster. Try to choose food products that indicate about 10 grams of fiber per 100 grams.

Sodium: If you think sugar and fat are dangerous components in your food, sodium is probably even worse, especially to those with cardiovascular health issues or hypertension. The American Heart Association advises that for an average 2000-calorie diet, we shouldn't eat more than 1500 milligrams of sodium a day. But if you look closely, many ready-made products like soups, TV dinners, and frozen foods, already contain a high level of sodium that can cause us to greatly exceed our daily sodium level. Try to choose products that contain less than 200 milligrams of sodium per every 100 grams. A product is considered low in sodium if it has .25 milligrams (mg) or less of salt per every 100 grams (or 100 milligrams of sodium or less per every 100 grams of the product).

Calcium: It is essential to keep our bones and muscles working properly, which is why it is recommended to choose products that contain more than 100 milligrams of calcium per every 100 grams.

Daily value or %DV: This number is a mystery to many, but it's really not that complicated! %DV stands for "Percent Daily Value" and indicates the nutritional intake of a portion of food for one person, based on the recommended 2000-calorie diet. If the product indicates 20% DV, it means the product provides 20% of the calories, carbohydrates, fiber, fat, etc., you need for one day if you're on a 2000-calorie diet. (Of course this is a very generic index, as it doesn't really translate to the individual needs of a child, a teenager who plays sports, an office worker who gets little exercise, a senior with limited mobility, etc., all of whom may need more or less than 2000 calories. Use %DV with caution!)

Below is a sample of a nutritional label. See how well you can decipher it!

Serving size: 1 cup or 100ml of milk

- Calories 45 kcal (g); 3.4g of protein; 1.5g fat; 4.6g carbohydrates; 20mg sodium; and 13g sugar

Vitamins and minerals the product contains in 100ml:

- Vitamin A 70 mg; Vitamin C 3.5 mg; Vitamin D 0.7 micrograms; Niacin 1.2 mg; Vitamin B6 0.1 mg; Folate 21 micrograms; Vitamin B12 0.1 micrograms; Calcium 120 mg; Phosphorus 95 mg; Iron 0.7 mg; Zinc 1.1 mg

SIX REASONS TO NOT COUNT CALORIES

Many people think that if you want to lose weight, you must count each of the calories you ingest. "Count your calories to lose weight" is a myth that has been repeated so often in so many spheres, many dieters swear by it. I'm here to tell you that keeping a food diary can help you lose weight, but obsessing over counting all the calories you eat may not be a good idea.

Here are six reasons why counting calories is not the one-size-fits-all answer to losing weight:

1. *The list of ingredients is more important than the number of calories.* Swapping a bag of chips for a pack of low-calorie crackers, doesn't mean that the crackers are "good" for you! These crackers could be filled with artificial ingredients to enhance their flavor. To lose weight, it is important to focus on the *quality* of the ingredients you eat, not the just the *quantity* of calories. It is crucial to always read the list of ingredients and their nutrition facts.

2. *Fewer calories are not always better.* Calorie-counting oversimplifies the complex world of health and nutrition. Choosing to eat a low-calorie diet instead of a healthy and balanced diet can lead to serious nutritional deficiencies, diseases, and disorders. It is very important to consider

the amounts of vitamins, minerals, enzymes and other nutrients from the foods we eat, and not just the calories!

3. *Eating shouldn't be mechanical.* When you limit yourself to a certain number of calories, you ignore the possibility that you are still hungry, even if you already ate the permissible amount of calories for that meal. It is essential to adopt a healthy attitude toward food. By eating slowly and with awareness, we'll develop a more harmonious relationship with the food on our plate, allowing it to nourish our cells. If you are always feeling hungry, even after hitting your "calorie quota," something might be wrong with your diet!

4. *Eating shouldn't increase your stress level.* As I mentioned before, stressing out about counting calories when you eat is not healthy for your body, especially your digestive health. It can mess up our metabolic response, which also promotes depression and anxiety, which can in turn affect some of our major organs, such as the stomach, liver, and pancreas. It could also keep our digestive system from properly absorbing the nutrients from the foods we eat.

5. *Not all calories are equal.* It is important to highlight that the calories from proteins, fats, and carbs are not all the same. Each one of them affects our metabolic rate, our hormones, and our appetite differently. For example, eating 100 calories of coconut oil will provide our body with quick energy. And because it is burned immediately by our body due to its short chain fatty acids, it also satisfies our appetite. But 100 calories of a protein shake are not absorbed the same way; it takes a lot longer to be digested and it may not be available for our body to use right away. In fact, additives and other lower quality ingredients you may find in these types of drinks could actually disrupt the normal functions of your system.

6. *The best foods don't have nutrition facts.* Without a doubt, the most complete foods are found in the fruits and vegetable section. These are nature's gift to us, and they don't come with a nutrition facts label. These are the most nutritious foods in the entire world. It is important to, as much as possible, avoid processed and pre-packaged foods. Fill your fridge with unpasteurized, raw foods, and many fruits and vegetables. And believe me when I tell you that, even if they are high in calories, you'll still be able to lose weight.

WHAT ABOUT PROTEIN POWDER?

Let's explore a few points here, because I get this question very often. First of all, let's explain what protein is. Protein is the main nutrient for muscle development in the body. Its presence and function are vital, because it is linked to all biological functions from the metabolism to the immune system. It helps you to lose weight without sacrificing muscle mass.

There are two kinds of protein: animal and vegetable. Animal proteins include eggs, poultry, fish, and meat and dairy products. Vegetable proteins include soybeans, beans and legumes, nuts, grains, and mushrooms. Below I've listed several good protein sources, along with the percentage of the product that is protein.

Animal Protein

- Monterey, low-fat Cheddar, or low-fat Colby cheese: 24% protein
- Tuna: 23% protein
- Chicken breast: 22.8% protein
- Turkey ham: 22.4% protein
- Canned sardines: 22% protein
- Lean beef: 21% protein
- Goat cheese: 21% protein
- Veal: 20.7% protein

- Grilled chicken: 20.6% protein
- Cow liver: 20.5% protein
- Salmon: 19% protein
- Lamb: 18% protein
- Cod: 17% protein
- Egg white: 11% protein
- Fat-free milk: 3.5% protein

Vegetable Protein

- Lentils: 23.5% protein
- Peas: 23% protein
- Chickpeas: 20% protein
- Almonds: 20% protein
- White beans: 19% protein
- Pistachios: 17.6% protein

Which is better? Nowadays, many people choose to lead a vegan or vegetarian lifestyle and they say that the "fewer legs" the source of protein has, the better. But in my experience, I feel that generally, except in cases of specific diseases, we need animal protein as well as vegetable protein.

How much protein should you eat? There is a lot of controversy regarding this question, and it is important to consider that the needs and conditions of each person are completely different. And, of course, before starting a new lifestyle, always consult with a specialist.

But generally speaking, a twenty-year-old woman, for example, requires approximately 38 grams of protein a day. If she is pregnant, it increases to around 50 grams, and if she is breast-feeding, around 60 grams.

There is also a basic table for us women to calculate the amount of protein we need according to our weight and within the context of being well-nourished. The formula is very easy: just multiply 0.36 times your weight in pounds. So, for example, if you weigh 145 pounds, multiply that number by 0.36. That equals to 52 grams of protein that you need daily. The minimum amount of protein for an adult woman to avoid health problems is her weight in pounds multiplied by 0.22.

Many women ask me if it's necessary to incorporate protein powder into their diet. My answer is that if your diet is providing the right amount of protein that your body needs, then you don't have to invest in a powdered protein.

But it so happens that sometimes it is very difficult to eat the amount of protein our body needs. Most of us today spend a lot of time away from home, working extremely long days, eating poorly, and spending many hours without eating a single bite of food. This makes us neglect the protein level we need, which is actually harmful to our health, especially if we maintain an exercise regimen at least three times a week.

In such cases, adding a protein shake to a healthy diet can be beneficial for us, especially after exercising. Doubling your protein intake from 2% to 4% can help build muscle mass. But don't imagine muscle like a bodybuilder's; rather, this builds the right type of muscle to show off strong legs and arms. It also helps you have a smaller percentage of body fat and increases lean muscle mass, which means better muscle tone and fewer problems like cellulite.

To return to one point I mentioned before: another huge benefit of protein is that it helps keep you satisfied for longer and accelerates your metabolism, two key parts to losing weight. For example, replacing one meal a day, such as a snack, with a protein shake instead, can be helpful. Protein powder also helps reduce the risk of osteoporosis, a condition that affects bone density in women, especially as we age.

For optimal absorption of protein shakes, you need to include foods that stimulate the production of hydrochloric acid such as spinach, kale, onions, garlic, and apple cider vinegar. Hydrochloric acid helps digest foods and proteins, since they are a bit more complex. It is best to eat these foods just before or after you drink your protein shake. And here's another helpful tip: bromelain is an enzyme supplement that can also help you with your digestion and the absorption of protein. The recommended daily dose is 500 milligrams.

Adding powdered protein to a healthy diet may also help lower cholesterol, blood pressure, and body mass faster than simply eating a healthy diet.

Here are a few more advantages of protein powders over protein in other forms:

+ They are digested and absorbed faster especially after exercise.
+ They provide a greater supply of amino acids.
+ They are easy and practical to take anywhere.

It is always a good idea to consult with your doctor before adding any supplements to your diet. If you suffer from kidney problems or diabetes, it is probably not a good idea to add protein powders to your diet. Also, people who suffer from reflux may find that too much protein in their diet worsens their digestive difficulties.

Some tips you should consider before buying a protein powder:

+ If you can, opt for a protein made of whey; it has a much more complete composition, in addition to better and more quickly absorbed amino acids.
+ Make sure that it is low in carbohydrates.
+ Make sure that it is low in sugar and doesn't contain artificial sweeteners.
+ It should contain at least 21 grams of protein per serving.
+ It should be low in sodium (no more than 60 milligrams).
+ If you're lactose intolerant, be aware that some protein powders contain milk products.

There are so many types and brands of protein powders on the market now, with different ingredients and formulas, that to find the ideal one for you is a complicated task. Here are a few info tips and facts to help you out.

ANIMAL PROTEIN POWDERS

Egg protein: It's of high quality and easy to digest. It contains over 40 different proteins, such as albumin, and others, like ovotransferrin, which contribute to iron binding. It's also rich in amino acids, including leucine, which helps stimulate protein synthesis, and arginine, which helps stimulate the production of nitric oxide, increasing blood flow to muscles, with more oxygen, nutrients, and anabolic hormones that elevate the energy level, improving performance and muscle recovery.

Whey protein: It's the most popular one because it is easy and quick to digest. It has a powerful antioxidant called glutathione along with an abundance of amino acids that reach the bloodstream quickly. It also increases the level of insulin, helps control cholesterol, and lowers blood pressure, because it dilates the blood vessels. According to the Mayo Clinic, "most studies suggest that whey protein increases feelings of fullness and reduces food intake."[2]

Casein protein: It comes from milk. It is not soluble in water and takes up to seven hours for our body to completely digest. It feeds the muscles much more than whey, but because of its complexity to digest, it is advisable to drink it at night before bed. A study by the University of Texas found that combining whey and casein protein considerably increases the development of muscle mass over drinking just the whey protein. But keep in mind that it is not recommended for those who are allergic or lactose intolerant or for those who have attention deficit disorder, epilepsy, or are sensitive to casein.

---

2. "Whey Protein Evidence," *Patient Care and Health Information*, Mayo Clinic, http://www.mayoclinic.org/drugs-supplements/whey-protein/evidence/hrb-20060532 (accessed September 30, 2015).

Goat whey protein: It contains casein and whey proteins like cow's milk, but the big difference is that its level of casein is lower, making it much friendlier for those who are allergic to dairy. Moreover, most of the brands are made from organic goat milk, which means no pesticides, herbicides, growth hormones, or antibiotics.

VEGETABLE PROTEIN

Brown rice protein: It has four times more arginine than whey protein and more than any other protein powder. Arginine is an essential amino acid for humans because, among other things, it contributes to the endocrine system and maintains the balance between nitrogen and carbon dioxide. It is of vital importance in the development of the growth hormone, the growth of tissues and muscles, and the maintenance and recovery of the immune and nervous systems, among other benefits.

Pea protein: It is a good alternative source of protein. It's also rich in arginine, with nearly three times more than whey protein. It contains significant amounts of glutamine, another essential amino acid. It is rich in BCAAs, or branched chain amino acids, which are essential to the immune system.

Hemp protein: Although it is in the same family as marijuana, its properties are completely different. It is a complete protein because it has the 10 essential amino acids and the 20 known ones. These include edestin and albumin, which puts it at the same level of egg protein. Edestin is necessary for a strong immune system to produce antibodies; while albumin helps maintain healthy liver and kidneys. This protein is also rich in arginine and BCAA.

TYPES OF FILTERING

Another aspect that we must consider when choosing a protein powder is the filtering process used to remove its fat, carbohydrates, and water.

Concentrated: When a shake is concentrated, it means that it has gone through minimal processing. It doesn't take away from its quality, but its digestion is medium to low.

Isolated: When a shake is isolated, it means it has been more filtered; it contains less fat and carbohydrates. Its digestion and absorption is faster than the protein concentrate.

Hydrolyzed: When a shake is hydrolyzed, it means that it has been even more filtered and made into a form available to be used as an amino acid. Its digestion and absorption is much faster than either concentrated or isolated shakes.

WHEN SHOULD YOU DRINK A PROTEIN SHAKE?

+ In the morning

After so many hours of fasting, your body is screaming for help in its recovery process. A protein shake that provides between 20 to 40 grams of fast digestion protein is an excellent choice.

+ Before training

A protein shake that contains about 20 grams of easily absorbed protein, like whey protein powder, about 30 minutes before exercising, can help you prepare the muscles to train as hard as possible. It also accelerates the muscle tissue recovery process.

+ After training

A shake that has 20 to 40 grams of fast-absorbing protein, about 30 minutes after exercising, helps maintain muscle recovery because it retains the amino acids, improving protein synthesis.

+ Between meals

Eating shakes as a snack is a perfect option because they will keep you satisfied until your next meal.

+ Before going to bed

Although we're resting, our metabolism continues to run and needs energy to do so. A slow-absorption protein shake helps stimulate the growth hormone that contributes to the formation of muscle tissue, preventing fat formation.

In a nutshell, it is very easy and convenient to add a few tablespoons to your morning smoothie to activate your metabolism 100%. But it is very important to keep in mind that protein powder should not replace a balanced diet in which you include plant and animal proteins. You should not rely solely on protein powders because your body does not digest them the same way it does foods. A balanced diet combined with a protein powder can supplement your needs and improve your performance, bump up your metabolism, and obtain better results. If you complement your healthy diet with regular exercise and the right protein shake, you can rest assured you'll see results sooner than you expect!

Chapter 4

CRAVINGS BE GONE!

When you get excited to change your life, you finally decide to get rid of those extra pounds! So you "jump in the water" of your weight-loss journey.

You start exercising and eating healthy. At first, everything works perfectly. You begin to see results, both in the mirror and on the scale. But just when you start to really get excited, thinking that you finally broke the barrier and have left behind all the suffering from weight gain, that's just when *it* rears its ugly head.

It destroys your progress! It sets you back! It steals your confidence!

What's *it*? Those monsters: food cravings! The pesky demons that terrorize dieters, robbing from us the results of our efforts because once they "bite" you, they mark the end of your journey. It doesn't matter how well you were doing. It doesn't matter how fierce your willpower. It doesn't even matter how badly you want to lose weight. Once those cravings take a hold of you, it becomes almost impossible to maintain a good diet.

Weeks and weeks of dieting and exercise are ruined in just a few days of rabidly eating ice cream, cookies, and any other sugary foods within reach.

Personally, my biggest problem was soda. No matter how hard I tried to stay away, the cravings were so intense that I always ended up falling into their claws. After the first sip, nothing could stop me.

I would drink five, seven, even ten sodas a day! I consumed hundreds and even thousands of empty calories. This caused the little bit of weight I had lost by dieting to come back faster than I could say *food craving*.

I knew that had to change. If I wanted to achieve my goals, I had to find a way to avoid those awful cravings. So pay attention because in the next few lines you will discover everything you need to know in order to eliminate those cravings, including the "trigger" foods. And you'll understand why that is the key to get rid of those extra pounds and inches.

I will also give tips and tricks to use when you feel those cravings are on their way, ready to attack. Turn your monster craving into a little kitty cat that will only do as you say!

It's time to get excited! Because once you put these techniques to work, you will be able to fight this major problem affecting your healthy diet. We can't leave anything to chance if we are taking our weight and health care seriously.

ADDICTIVE TRIGGER FOODS THAT CAUSE MASSIVE CRAVINGS

Have you ever felt "defeated" by a craving? And I don't mean that you *want* to eat something; I mean that you feel you *have* to eat it or you'll die. You feel that you just couldn't carry on with your life or feel satisfied until you eat it.

We've all been there, right? It happens when there is absolutely no willpower, when we don't care how bad the food is for us and our health—because it feels like our body is just screaming for it.

Well, it turns out that those cravings, which can destroy our efforts, are not only in our head. The reason we feel we have to eat and that it is impossible to stop once we start is because these foods are highly addictive!

These foods are called "trigger foods" and their effect on our brain is similar to a drug or alcohol effect. They stimulate the reward center of the brain, releasing endorphins that make us feel good—and can be addictive.

We begin to associate feelings of pleasure with these foods, and the connection can be so strong that we can begin to release endorphins such as dopamine *just by thinking of them!*

It has been shown that dopamine improves our consciousness and increases the feeling of pleasure, so once the body starts pumping it, the cravings are impossible to forget.

So, what do we do?

Well, the most common mistake people make is to say that they'll just have "a little" to satisfy the craving and then go on with their day.

Big mistake.

When you eat these foods, your body produces a physical response that makes you want more and more. Once you start, it is impossible to stop, and that "little bit" turns into compulsive face-stuffing. The only way to prevent this is by recognizing which foods produce this response in your body. Once you identify them, you'll be able to avoid them, rather than getting stuck in their claws. We need to know our enemy.

So let's talk about these "trigger" foods.

TRIGGER FOOD #1: SUGAR

If you really want to lose weight, then sugar is the worst thing that you can give to your body. When you eat sugar, the body releases a hormone called insulin. Insulin is known as the storage hormone. When insulin levels in your body are high, you store fat instead of burning it for energy. When you eat too much sugar, your insulin levels remain high, making it almost impossible to burn fat!

But this is not the worst part. Sugar can be extremely addictive—brain scan studies have shown that the addictive effects of sugar are similar to those of cocaine! You see, when you eat sugar, your body releases endorphins that make you feel like you're "high." But to keep that effect, you have to eat more and more sugar. You begin to depend on sugar as a real drug.

Also, when you eat sugar, your body releases another hormone called ghrelin, which is known as the hunger hormone. This stimulates your appetite even more, making those cravings worse.

Finally, sugar creates a "memory storage" in your body. Your body remembers the good feeling it got from eating sugar. The more memories you create (eating sugar), the stronger your sugar cravings will be in the future.

If you are willing to lose weight, you have to avoid processed sugar—and I'm also referring to white flour because, once it's in the body, it gets converted into sugar. Once you avoid it for long enough, you'll see that those cravings for ice cream, candy, and cookies, among many others, begin to disappear.

TRIGGER FOOD #2: CHOCOLATE

Chocolate affects the body very similarly to sugar, which makes sense because they go hand in hand. When you eat chocolate, your body releases serotonin, a chemical that makes you "feel good" and is responsible for your good mood.

The only problem is that to stay in a good mood, you have to eat more and more chocolate. This can increase your cravings, making them more intense. Chocolate also contains caffeine and theobromine, stimulants that can add to the addictive effects. And because chocolate is so high in calories, it is not something you want to get addicted to when trying to lose weight.

TRIGGER FOOD #3: CHEESE

Cheese is another food very high in calories, and it is very hard to stop eating it. You always start with a little bit, but before you know it, you've eaten everything in front of you!

There is a simple explanation why cheese is so addictive, and you may be surprised to know the reason why. Cheese has a milk protein called casein. When digested, your body breaks it down into particles containing morphine. Yes, morphine, the same drug that is given to patients in extreme pain. So if you find yourself eating cheese like a mouse, you now know why!

TRIGGER FOOD #4: GREASY FOOD

If you find yourself craving fatty foods, is not only because they are delicious. This goes deeper. Foods high in saturated fats like bacon or red meat toy with your body's ability to withstand cravings and control your appetite.

When you eat these types of foods, you will eat until you are completely full. By then, it's too late. You've already overeaten. But the problem is not overeating once. The effect that these foods have on your appetite can last up to three days, because that's the time it takes your body to remove all the fat from the system. Until then, the cravings will keep coming again and again.

Also, red meat contains a stimulant called hypoxanthine. It's what causes that satisfying feeling you get after eating a good steak. And once it's in your system, it can make you feel like you're missing something unless you eat more meat.

TRIGGER FOOD #5: CORN

You probably say you never eat corn, meaning that you never put a corn cob at your table or garnish your plate with corn kernels. You have no idea, however, that you are eating it in a thousand different ways because it is found in almost all foods in your menu, adding hundreds of calories and dozens of hidden carbohydrates to your diet. Even if you've never had corn on the cob or ever tried corn oil, you are still eating it in excess during the day because corn is in almost everything we eat.

This ingredient messes up your blood sugar, increases your insulin levels, and causes your body to store all the fat.

In some foods, it is used as a filling; a "cheap" way to extend the shelf life of the product in the supermarket. In other foods, it's used as a sweetener known as high fructose corn syrup; a simple carbohydrate that elevates insulin, very similarly to table sugar, preventing your body from burning fat for energy.

If you eat foods that come in a box or bag such as cereal, salad dressings, fruit juices, ketchup, jams, sauces, frozen foods, soft drinks and ice cream, then all you have to do is read the label on these foods to find this ingredient that makes you fat.

But even if you avoid junk food, even if your diet is filled with whole foods, that doesn't mean you're safe from eating corn. You can even find it in beef! Most cattle are raised on a grain-based diet. The most common feeding ingredient is corn. So now we eat it every time we put a steak on a grill or bake a chicken.

Although corn is cheaper for farmers, it reduces the quality of the meat. Cows are born to eat grass. When you feed them grains, they develop health problems; to stay healthy, they are treated with harmful antibiotics that are then transferred to us through the meat we eat. Grain-fed beef is low in omega-3 fatty acids, the healthy kind we need to enjoy great cardiovascular and mental health.

It's not hard to see the consequences of this problem. It is not hard to understand how the presence of corn in our diet makes losing weight a difficult task. All this is easy to see and understand, but the solution to the problem may be a bit more complicated.

First of all, you need to eliminate all processed foods from your diet. Soft drinks, fruit juices, cakes, cookies, and, well, anything that contains high fructose corn syrup, should be avoided as much as possible. Instead, eat fresh natural foods like fruits and vegetables.

Second, the best thing to do is to eat meat from grass-fed cows. Yes, it is a bit more expensive, but the impact it has on our health is worth it. If you need motivation, just don't forget that all those carbohydrates end up on your waistline—and then you'll be spending money to lose the weight!

BE CAREFUL WITH SALT

So far so good; but before finishing with this section, I have to mention one harmful ingredient that, even after you eliminate all the ones I mentioned above, still has the potential to hinder your efforts.

Let's say you don't eat sugar, you completely eliminate corn and fatty foods, and you are following all of the tricks I gave you. However, you're still not losing weight. Does this sound familiar? If so, then it's probably because you're consuming too much sodium.

That's right, salt is an ingredient found in each one of our meals that makes it almost impossible to lose weight. We've already talked about how sugar, like simple carbs, is a big enemy when trying to lose weight, because sugar sends fat-storing signals to your body. We've also noted the negative impact the wrong kinds of fats have on our health. And now we are going to focus on those little white magical grains that are even more addictive...and just as dangerous, if not more dangerous.

Sodium dehydrates us; it causes difficulty in breathing and forces our heart to work harder. And even if you do not know it, the chances of consuming *excess* sodium are very high, because most people believe that by only eliminating table salt, they are eliminating it completely from their diets. But it's not as simple as that! Sodium is hidden in most foods we eat.

It is found in meat, fish, and seafood. It's even in milk! Although these products are not full of sodium, the sodium level starts to add up gradually. And it can lead us to consume more than we should in a day. This becomes a big problem for our diet!

All processed foods are full of sodium. This includes pizza, pasta, potato chips, cereal, bacon, ham, processed cheeses, fast foods; sodium is even in whey protein powders and bars! So basically, if the food product comes in a box or bag, most probably, it has more sodium than is good for you.

Sodium is added to food as a preservative so that it has a longer shelf life. Canned and boxed foods contain lots of sodium; companies use this method to reduce their production costs and sell more. Our health is not their top priority!

Now, don't misunderstand me. Sodium is not bad for you. Our bodies need a certain amount to function properly. It is an important mineral, but like everything else, sodium must be consumed in moderation. There must be a balance for an easier weight-loss journey.

Unfortunately, the foods we eat often dangerously increase the levels of sodium in our bodies. If you regularly eat fast food or junk food, chances are that your health is in danger.

You don't believe me? Read these statistics:

A very popular chain restaurant in the United States, was sued due to the incredible amount of sodium that they added to their meals. Moreover, it was shown that their scrambled eggs, "Meat Lovers," which is a popular breakfast in their more than 1,500 restaurants, contained 5,690 milligrams of sodium. That's almost the recommended amount of sodium to be consumed by an adult—in a three-day period!

It is incredible! There are other restaurants, just as popular as this fast food chain, that are great examples of how we put our health at risk by eating their meals.

It's no joke.

If you consume excess sodium, your blood pressure rises, making your kidneys work harder than their optimum level to lower sodium levels in the blood. And when there is too much to eliminate, the sodium just begins to accumulate. From the kidneys, it goes to the arteries, where it could cause blockage, making our heart overwork and eventually, leading to heart failure.

It also makes us look horrible! Sodium produces excessive dehydration. Absorbing the water from our cells, this water gets trapped beneath the skin, somehow making it really difficult for our body to use it, so we begin to feel the effects of dehydration such as thirst, lack of energy, and a dry mouth. And since the water is trapped underneath our skin, we look bloated.

Our body begins to retain all the extra water, and we can notice this in the mirror and the scale. And none of us can get rid of this situation!

There was one time when I was at a conference that I simply had no time to eat, let alone find some healthy food. I just grabbed whatever was in sight from the food that they offered. What was the result? I gained six pounds!

I didn't panic, because I knew that my body is a sophisticated calculating machine, and if I returned to the correct input, it would result in my normal body weight, which is exactly what happened. However, it taught me to be much more careful about the decisions I make when I travel.

So what can we do to stay in the healthy sodium range? Well, there is a simple two-step process to do so.

First, stay away from table salt. Don't count on it to add flavor to your foods; instead, there are tons of spices you can use to add flavor without jeopardizing your health, such as garlic, rosemary, thyme, onion, paprika, and dill. These are all great alternatives to salt.

Second, you have to eliminate processed foods from your diet; avoid foods like cakes, cookies, potato chips and boxed cereal, among many others. You also have to reduce your fast food consumption. Focus on natural, fresh, and homemade foods such as lean meats, fruits, vegetables, whole foods, and whole grains, among others.

As long as you eat this way, you'll see your sodium levels begin to decline naturally. And you will begin to lose all the retained liquids in your body.

So be sure to control your sodium intake and you'll see amazing results!

I'm also going to ask you to please share this information with your friends and family. The effects of excess sodium are very dangerous. Remember: excessive sodium intake is a mistake we all can make. There are many mistakes that can prevent us from losing weight and deteriorate our health; mistakes you probably don't even know you are making.

Remember that the small but horrible monsters of sugar, chocolate, cheese, corn, and fatty foods, are the real culprits of your uncontrollable cravings. By avoiding them, you will be able to control your weight more easily.

But if one of them crosses your path, the nine tricks and tips I'll share with you next can save you from falling into the trap!

ELIMINATE YOUR SUGAR CRAVINGS WITH THESE 9 "CRAVING KICKERS"

As long as you stay away from the "trigger foods" that I mentioned, you will find that those awful cravings will start to disappear.

Eventually, you'll build momentum for your mind and body, and you'll be able to eat these foods without losing control. But sometimes, avoiding them is not enough. Sometimes, you feel a craving coming and you know that if you fall for it, you will trigger a chain reaction of bad decisions that will keep you away from the good results you want.

Don't let that happen! You need to make those cravings disappear quickly. By using these tricks, you'll be able to make it.

Give it a try...

CRAVING KICKER #1: EAT MORE FREQUENT AND SMALLER PORTIONS THROUGHOUT THE DAY.

This strategy helps keep your metabolism active so you can burn fat twenty-four hours a day. But it also helps prevent cravings.

Many times, cravings are a way for the body to say that it's hungry. If you go too long without eating, your body will have cravings. Processed foods are usually full of sugar, and they are the fastest way to solve the problem. So when you feel hungry, that is what the body craves.

But if you eat in small portions during the day, you'll keep the body nourished. Sugar levels stay balanced, and you won't get those horrible desires to devour everything.

CRAVING KICKER #2: INCLUDE PROTEIN IN EVERY MEAL.

Protein is one of the best things you can eat when you want to lose weight. Since it takes a long time for the body to digest, it gives you a satiating effect. It can keep you full and satisfied for longer periods of time, making you less likely to fall into the trap of cravings. Some examples of protein-rich foods are chicken, turkey, fish, eggs, nuts, legumes, and tofu.

CRAVING KICKER #3: AVOID SUGAR AT BREAKFAST.

In the first section, we discussed the addictive effects of sugar. We said that if you eat sugar, your body releases endorphins that make you feel good. And to keep this good mood you're in, you have to eat more and more sugar. We also talked about how eating sugar causes a hormone called ghrelin to be released and stimulate your appetite.

All these things happen when you eat sugar. And guess what most people do? They begin their day with a breakfast full of sugar—eating cereals, doughnuts, bread, and biscuits, among others. These common breakfast foods are loaded with sugar and when you eat them, you put yourself in a position to suffer from cravings for the entire day.

That's why you should avoid a sugar-filled breakfast. Eat protein-rich foods in the morning. Eggs, yogurt, or a protein shake will help you to avoid spending the day suffering from cravings.

CRAVING KICKER #4: AVOID ARTIFICIAL SWEETENERS.

Many people consider "diet" drinks to be a good alternative for sugar. They think that as long as they change that soda to its "diet" version, they can have all the soda they want. Unfortunately, that is not how it works.

The artificial sweeteners that are used in these diet drinks also cause cravings. When you drink them, you trick your body. It detects the sweet taste and expects sugar. Then, when the sugar never arrives, your body "craves" it even more.

That is why artificial sweeteners are terrible when you're dieting. Although the product may say "calorie free," that doesn't mean it's "craving free!" In fact, it's basically saying, "guaranteed to increase craving by 100%!"

Avoid diet drinks; drink water instead. Jamaican water and oolong tea are excellent choices to stay hydrated and to refresh (more on that in chapter 5!). If you need something sweet, make some green tea and add a little Stevia. It tastes great with ice.

CRAVING KICKER #5: DISTRACT YOUR MIND.

The worst thing you can do when you have a craving is to sit down and think about it. Next time you get one, you can eliminate it by occupying your mind with something else. Go for a walk, run errands, clean your house, read a book—it doesn't matter what you do, just do something! When you are busy, you don't have the mental energy to think about unhealthy foods.

CRAVING KICKER #6: WASH DOWN YOUR CRAVINGS.

This is one of the simplest things you can do. It is also one of the most effective. The next time you feel a craving coming, drink a large glass of water. Most of the time, you'll feel those cravings disappear.

Why does this happen? Many times, when we feel hunger, it is the body saying it is dehydrated. Sometimes it is hard to tell the difference between the two, and since food also contains water, it is a simple way for the body to get the water it needs. But you can eliminate that "fake hunger" faster by having a glass of water.

So next time you are craving unhealthy foods, before you grab that bag of chocolates, drink a glass of water and wait to see if those cravings disappear.

Most often, they will!

CRAVING KICKER #7: CLEAN TEETH EQUALS NO CRAVINGS.

This is one of my favorite tricks to eliminate cravings. When you feel a craving coming, stop whatever you are doing and go brush your teeth!

It sounds strange, but it works because if you brush your teeth and have that clean feeling in your mouth, you tend to want to keep it. You don't want to ruin it by chewing sugary foods.

So by keeping your mouth clean and fresh, you can keep away that "sweet tooth." (Not to mention that it's great for dental hygiene!)

CRAVING KICKER #8: EAT FRUIT.

If you still feel like eating something sweet, then eat fruit. It will help you satisfy your craving and the natural sugars the fruit contains also come with vitamins and minerals that are good for your health.

The best thing to do is to avoid falling into the trap of your cravings, using tricks 1–7, because it is not good for your mind to accept defeat. But having some fruit occasionally will not hurt.

CRAVING KICKER #9: KEEP FRESHLY CUT VEGGIES HANDY.

Carrots and celery are a good alternative to whatever you're craving. Carrying a bag of them with you can be a great help when cravings strike, because the crunch from the fresh veggies can help distract your mind, and the fiber content satisfies your need to eat.

Chapter 5

CHUG, CHUG, CHUG!

If you are eating healthily and exercising regularly, and still don't see the results that you want to see on the scale (and the mirror), the information that I am about to share with you can give you the boost that you need.

Eating the right foods is not enough. It is a good start, but the food is only half of what you consume.

The other half comes from what you drink. If you are like most people, what you drink is making it almost impossible for you to get the body that you would die for! If we fill up with sugary drinks, those empty calories can put a "stop" sign on our weight-loss efforts. In fact, drinking all those calories is a waste because you are ruining your efforts of eating healthily.

Ordering a salad with chicken instead of that burger or pizza is a worthless sacrifice if you're drinking a soda with it! Before drinking to quench your thirst, you must know that making the wrong decision about what you drink will quickly ruin your hopes of losing weight!

So, let's do this!

DRINKS TO AVOID

What are the wrong choices to drink? What drinks should you avoid to look great next summer?

First of all:

SUGARY DRINKS

You have to avoid all sugary drinks. This includes sodas, sports drinks, iced tea, and all sugary fruit juices.

All those drinks are filled with calories that turn into sugar. This spikes your insulin levels, wreaks havoc on your blood sugar levels, and is easily stored as fat.

DIET DRINKS

Don't think that you can drink beverages that say "light," "sugar free," or "diet." Even though there is less sugar in these drinks, they are still filled with toxic, artificial sweeteners to make them taste sweet. They also increase your sugar cravings, which make it more difficult to eat healthily.

COFFEE

I know that I'm about to break some hearts, but *stop drinking coffee*.

I'm sorry! I used to drink my cup of coffee every day, and I was really sad when I realized that I had to quit. However, after three weeks, I didn't even miss it. I learned to substitute my cup of coffee for a cup of oolong tea. In fact, I drink it during the day and today, it is my favorite drink. Oolong tea is completely natural; it is rich in vitamins and antioxidants that provide me with more energy. I feel more relaxed and rejuvenated all day long.

The caffeine found in coffee is a stimulant that acts on the central nervous system; the "high" is followed by a depressive stage, ending in fatigue, nervousness, irritability, and often a headache.

You also want to avoid drinking caffeinated drinks. This includes not just coffee, but other energy drinks (that are often filled with sugar). These drinks put stress on your adrenal glands and dehydrate you, which makes it difficult to lose weight. Yes, I know these drinks provide you with a boost of energy, but they are always followed by an energy crash.

So, do you think that experiencing these side effects is worth it?

ALCOHOLIC BEVERAGES

You should also avoid alcoholic beverages. I know that this is something that you do not want to hear, and drinking occasionally may be fine, but *not* while you are trying to lose weight. Alcohol not only dehydrates you; it impairs your judgment and increases your cravings for unhealthy foods. Also, a lot of the mixers used for "mixed drinks" are almost entirely made up of sugar, which we already know sends our bodies into fat storage mode.

It is one of the worst things that you can put in your body if you are trying to lose weight. Let me quickly explain why, in easy bullet-point format:

+ It is filled with sugar.
+ It impairs your judgment and willpower to stay away from unhealthy foods.
+ It increases your appetite, making you eat anything, even if it is not healthy.
+ It causes dehydration. When your body is dehydrated, it is prone to store fat.
+ It causes depression, which makes you eat in a compulsive way.

✦ It causes lack of concentration and energy.

Don't you think it is a good idea to avoid it during your transformation?

I would love to sit down and give you a list of cocktails, beers, and wines that are healthier, but the fact is that they are all bad for you. I don't recommend any alcoholic beverage, for at least the first 21 days of your new eating habits.

If you can wait 21 years to start drinking, you can wait 21 days to break the habit.

You will lose weight by not going to happy hour or girls' night out. I lost fourteen pounds in 21 days! Once the three weeks have passed and you realize that you didn't really miss drinking alcohol, you will continue to lose weight.

SO, WHAT CAN I DRINK?

OOLONG TEA

Let's begin with my personal favorite: oolong tea! It will make you start your day filled with energy. It is a great substitute for coffee. Besides being delicious, it curbs your sugar cravings, helps you to lose weight, and has been shown to increase your body's fat burning rate by 35–43%. It's also been proven to burn up to 2 times more calories than green tea, which is also well-known for its weight-loss effects.

The only problem I ran into was that it is not easy to find a high-quality oolong tea! But God put somebody in my path who happened to own a manufacturer of high quality teas in China. He approached me to represent his brand, and our cooperation resulted in me being able to create my own brand of high-quality oolong tea. If you would like to know more about this tea and its benefits, I invite you to visit www.IMOolong.com.

HIBISCUS TEA

Another fantastic drink is hibiscus tea, also known as "Jamaican Water." It comes from a flower of the hibiscus tree. It is loaded with nutrients, and it has a naturally fruity flavor. It has been shown to lower blood pressure, as well as abdominal cramping, giving you a slimmer waist.

It's filled with Vitamin C, which helps boost your immune system. It is also filled with antioxidants that help the body combat illnesses, such as cancer. It is rich in electrolytes, making it ideal for your body to recover after working out. Electrolytes help muscles recover, eliminate excess water, and regulate blood acid levels.

Jamaican water alleviates menstrual cramps, normalizes blood pressure levels, cleanses your kidneys and arteries, and purifies and lowers cholesterol.

It is a great weight-loss ally because it is a natural diuretic, helping the body to eliminate toxins through the urine. It also inhibits enzymes that break down sugars and complex carbohydrates. A body free of toxins is a healthy body, and a healthy body enables weight loss.

WARM LEMON WATER

Don't be fooled by the simplicity of the recipe. It's one of the best things you can put in your body. Start your day with a glass of warm water and a squirt of lemon (or lime). This will work wonders on your health. The combination stimulates your kidneys and helps purify them from toxins. It has been shown that warm water and lemon help kidneys produce more healthy enzymes than any other food or drink. And with your kidneys working properly, you will be able to eliminate toxins from your fat cells, letting you burn fat a lot quicker.

But this is just the beginning. Warm water with lemon aids digestion. It also helps you maintain constant movement in your intestines, avoiding any "clogs."

Warm water and lemon is also very rich with important minerals. It is loaded with potassium, which is responsible for maintaining your immune system health. Low levels of potassium are linked to depression, anxiety, and forgetfulness. Warm water and lemon is rich in calcium, magnesium, and other important minerals that help maintain your bones and a healthy heart.

Warm water and lemon is one of the best sources of vitamin C and a powerful antioxidant that does wonders on your skin, helping to eliminate wrinkles and some imperfections. Vitamin C is one of the first nutrients that run out when you are stressed; so to avoid gaining weight due to your high stress levels, you must maintain high levels of Vitamin C. Vitamin C also keeps your immune system strong, keeping you free from illnesses that can rob you of your energy.

Even though many people know the effects of lemon, very few understand how it can help them lose weight. This may just be the most powerful effect that this "magical drink" has on the body. Water with lemon is not only a good source of incredible nutrients that increase your energy but can also help you control your appetite, which helps to burn fat.

And because this drink contains many minerals, it has an alkaline effect on the body, which helps neutralize acids. When your body has high levels of acid, it is hard for it to lose weight because it is not releasing any fat cells (remember that they are called "fatty acids" for a reason). So, the more acid is neutralized, the faster your body will be able to get rid of stored fat, letting you lose weight.

COCONUT WATER

Coconut water stays in your body longer than regular water, and it is more hydrating than energy and sports drinks. It is also an excellent way to keep you healthier. It is rich with potassium and low in sodium, which helps control high blood pressure. Coconut water is rich in essential electrolytes, such as magnesium, calcium, bicarbonate, and sulphate. It is natural and additive-free. It works as a natural diuretic, and it is cholesterol-free. The sugar found in it is completely natural; it also provides a little protein and vitamins.

If these benefits are not enough for you to want to try this drink, then consider the flavor. It is a sweet and thirst-quenching drink. It has been linked to weight loss. It is ideal for anybody with clean eating habits!

I love the fact that I can substitute it for all sports drinks. I was never a big fan of them anyway, because they are high in sugar, and they really didn't give me any energy during my workouts. I also love the fact that it hydrates me quickly, and the hydration lasts for a long time.

Keep in mind that there are different coconut water flavors, so their nutrients will also be different. Some flavors are higher in sugar than others. Just check the label and make sure there aren't any artificial additives. Taste it in your morning shakes. My favorite shake recipe is coconut water, spinach, kale, lemon juice, and apples. I call this shake "Lili," and I usually drink it in the mornings after working out to hydrate my body fast. Trust me, try it! Your family will love the flavor and its nutritional value.

COLD WATER

Water is a drink that your body needs—this shouldn't come as a surprise, since our bodies are made of 55–75% water. Besides oxygen, water is the most important nutrient to keep us alive. Our body uses water in almost every vital process. It aids digestion. It helps to regulate our body temperature. It keeps our joint articulations flexible and lubricated.

It also aids in the toxin elimination process. What will probably interest you even more is that it helps to get rid of body fat! You see, when you exercise, your body breaks down the stored fat. But after the fat has been broken down, your body produces by-products that need to be eliminated. Water will help you get rid of these.

Water and only water will be able to do this. Coffee, tea, sodas, and fruit juices are not good substitutes for it. Your body requires pure and natural water to stay hydrated and to eliminate toxins. When your body doesn't get enough water, the dehydration effects are felt right away. Your energy levels crash. You start to crave food. Yes, your body gets confused between being hungry and being thirsty. When you are not drinking enough water, you may feel hungry, and this could be a disaster when you are trying to lose weight.

But this is not the only thing that water does; studies have shown that by simply drinking eight glasses of cold water per day, you'll burn an extra 7.3 pounds of fat per year! It makes sense when you think about it: because the water that you are drinking is ice cold, before your body can use it, it needs to bring it up to room temperature. Heating this water requires energy and to get that energy, your body has to burn calories. Water is not only calorie-free (compared to the hundreds of calories found in a glass of soda), but it also makes your body *burn* calories when you drink it!

The reasons why you should drink eight glasses of water a day (preferably cold) are very clear. Avoid drinking coffee and sodas, and focus on drinking water instead! You will not only see your energy levels increase, but you will also see your body shed those extra pounds.

Do not underestimate the importance of liquids when it comes to your looks. When eliminating all those unhealthy and empty calories, you are giving your body the boost it needs to lose weight and finally turn into the sexy and slim body that you want!

GREEN TEA AND LEMON

Green tea stimulates the metabolism and boosts weight loss due to the powerful antioxidants content. Epigallocatechin gallate (EGCG), along with caffeine, stimulate the central and nervous systems, releasing the fat into the bloodstream, for the body to use as energy. This process, where the fat is used as energy, is called "thermogenesis." It provides you with extra energy; it gets rid of extra water; and it burns body fat, especially when you exercise for a long time.

Green tea also helps prevent the body from absorbing the fat from the foods that you eat. It optimizes your blood sugar levels and reduces cravings. It burns fat so your muscles stay strong. Even when you have reached your ideal weight, you should still enjoy green tea and all its long-term benefits, including its high antioxidant level and metabolism-boosting properties. And remember, green tea has less caffeine than coffee and regular teas, which makes it less harmful to your health.

Add lemon to this amazing drink and enjoy all of its added benefits, too. If you can't find oolong tea, remember that green tea can be a great option too.

MINT INFUSIONS TO BURN FAT

Mint tea stimulates gastric functions, increasing the digestive metabolism; it also acts on the gall bladder, stimulating and increasing bile secretion. It has the power to emulsify fat. It is rich with vitamin B, and it is a powerful anti-inflammatory.

It is a very refreshing and thirst-quenching drink. It has been shown to prevent bloating, because it helps to quickly digest the fat from the food, helping you slim down your belly.

The hardest thing that I had to do to get in shape was taking control of my bad drinking habits. But if you consciously make this change, it will be worth it. A little trick that I used to get into the habit of drinking water was to drink it with a straw. Drinking water from a colorful bottle with a straw, and carrying it around wherever you go, can help you to start drinking more water. It really works, trust me!

Chapter 6

THE TRICK TO GETTING A FLAT TUMMY...FAST!

Ugh! Abdominal fat. There is absolutely nothing that can ruin a woman's self-esteem more than extra pounds around her waist. It keeps you miles away from wearing the clothes that you love. It can make something as simple as taking a picture a total nightmare because you have to find the right angle that hides all the "imperfections."

Believe me, I know what it feels like. Before my 50-pound transformation, all I wished for was a flat stomach. However, it didn't matter how strict my diet was or how much I exercised, I simply couldn't get rid of my abdominal fat.

You see, abdominal fat is quite tricky because it's influenced by your hormone levels. If your hormone levels are out of control, it doesn't matter what you do, you will never get rid of it. On the other hand, if you are able to control your hormone levels, your fat will be able to disappear.

So, how do you do it?

Well, there are three things you must know.

SLEEP

First, you have to make sure you sleep at least seven hours, every night. It's funny because when you think about losing weight, you think about being active. But sometimes, the best thing to do for our body is to give it what it needs: sleep!

It has been shown that lack of sleep leads to weight gain. It makes us insulin-resistant, which kicks our bodies into fat-storing mode. It also controls leptin levels, a hormone known as the hunger hormone. So, if we don't get a good night's sleep, we will crave food more than usual, making it hard to lose weight.

And, as you must know from experience if you're anything like me, not having enough sleep can determine our mood the next day. Lack of sleep leads to a bad mood, fatigue, and irritability—just to name a few. It's highly likely that if you don't have a good night's sleep, your day will be compromised by your inability to pay attention and your constant yawning.

However, sleeping is not only important for your mood; it is also necessary to get good weight-loss results and be more efficient at the gym. When you are sleeping, your body releases high levels of the growth hormones that help to build muscle. It is also the only time when your muscles rest, which they desperately need because they are in constant movement and are constantly being stretched, especially during your workout routines.

Not sleeping enough also makes your body produce more cortisol, a chemical substance (a mix of high blood sugar levels and insulin levels). When your body detects cortisol, it gets confused and thinks it's hungry. Cortisol stores fat around the abdominal area. If you produce more of it, there is a chance that you are also storing more fat in your abdomen area.

So if you are sleepy and cranky, with a slow metabolism and increased hunger—wow, think about all the trouble you can get yourself into with that combination!

STRESS

Second, you have to reduce your stress levels. Stress not only wears us down mentally, it also has a negative impact on our bodies. It can lead us to suffer from heart difficulties, increase our blood pressure, and as you probably know, keep us from reaching our weight-loss goals.

When you have high stress levels, your body also produces cortisol, and it sends signals to your brain, telling it to store the most amount of fat possible. So, until you get your stress levels under control, you will have a hard time getting a thin waist.

SUPER FOODS

Finally, you have to include foods that fight fat. Every day.

Reducing the caloric intake is not enough. If you want a sexy and flat stomach, you have to eat foods that give your metabolism a boost and balance out your hormone levels. These foods are filled with proteins and are rich in fiber.

Fiber, protein, and good fats are essential in a daily food plan in order to have a flat tummy. These nutrients are found in these three super foods: wheat germ, chia seeds, and flaxseed. These three foods are rich in amino acids, proteins, and fatty acids such as omega-3 and fiber, all of which are essential to our body because they work toward eliminating the toxins and body fat that show in our abdomen.

On the other hand, it is very important to snack between meals. Eating every three to four hours will help you keep your blood sugar levels steady. A lot of people think that eating less will help reduce fat, but the reality is that going over four hours without eating will cause you to *gain* abdominal fat.

The best time to eat a snack, filled with proteins and fiber, is between 3:00 and 4:00 p.m. Snacking at this time is a *must*. A healthy afternoon munch will accelerate your metabolism and regulate your blood sugar levels. Remember, the lower your blood sugar level, the lower your insulin level, and the less fat around your stomach.

I am going to reveal a list of "super foods" that you can use to lose weight and get the body of your dreams. When you make these foods a part of your daily food plan, you make it easier to lose those unwanted pounds. Without wasting any more time, let's talk about them.

FOOD #1: OATMEAL

This one is perfect for breakfast.

As you may know, breakfast is the most important meal of the day. It gives our metabolism a boost to keep working during the day. You just need to eat the right breakfast.

You will never go wrong with oatmeal. This is the first choice for breakfast that sports enthusiasts prefer. It contains complex carbohydrates that fill you up with a long-lasting energy. Oatmeal is also rich in fiber, which is excellent for a good digestion, and it also helps you control your appetite in a natural way which means that you will be less likely to eat in excess.

FOOD #2: EGGS

Eggs are another delicious option for breakfast.

They are filled with complete proteins, vitamins, and minerals. Leucine is one of the amino acids found in eggs and is very beneficial for weight loss. It helps you keep a lean muscle, while it burns fat. I love to add mushrooms and bell peppers to make a delicious omelet filled with proteins and fibrous carbohydrates. Don't forget that the fiber helps you control your appetite.

FOOD #3: GRAPEFRUIT

This refreshing citrus has an incredible flavor and is very low in calories, making it ideal for a snack. It is filled with antioxidants that fight cancer, such as lycopene. It also helps your body respond better to insulin, a hormone that causes your body to store fat. This is very important; studies show that eating half of a grapefruit before your meals helps you lose weight!

FOOD #4: BERRIES

These little, tasty super foods are ideal for weight loss. They are filled with antioxidants that fight fat, helping keep your immune system healthy and your body and metabolism working at full speed.

Berries are so versatile. You can enjoy them alone, in a fruit salad, or you can blend them (with a scoop of whey protein) to create a delicious shake.

FOOD #5: AVOCADO

This is a very interesting fruit—yes, it is a *fruit*, and a great one for weight loss!

Avocados are delicious and nutritious. They contain an amino acid called L-carnitine that boosts your metabolism and accelerates your weight loss. Thanks to these incredible benefits, avocados should be included in the daily food plan of those trying to lose weight.

FOOD #6: RAW MACA POWDER

It comes from a root in Peru and is from the mustard family. It has been used for medicinal purposes, but it is great for your overall health. It is known to increase energy, fight against illnesses, improve your mood and immune system, and boost sexual function. It comes in powder and you can use it to make delicious and nutritious protein shakes. It has a nutty flavor that I think is incredibly tasty!

FOOD #7: GOJI BERRIES

If you want to boost your shake, you should add goji berries. These berries are a red-orange color and are native to China. They have been around for centuries, but have only recently become more popular in the Western world. They are filled with antioxidants and are known for their age-fighting attributes.

FOOD #8: SPIRULINA

Our next food comes from the lake. Spirulina is a small algae that grows in fresh water and for ages it has been known as *the* major healthy food. It is incredibly nutritious, filled with proteins, essential fats, vitamins, and minerals. This is what makes it so special—letting all its nutrients work together to broaden its vitality.

FOOD #9: CHIA SEEDS

This super food was mentioned on both *Oprah* and *Dr. Oz*, and for a good reason. Chia seeds are filled with nutrients and they are incredibly powerful for weight loss. They are filled with antioxidants, vitamins, fiber, omega-3 fatty acids, and minerals. They are a great source of complete protein that provide all the essential amino acids and are easy to digest. Chia seeds help to grow healthy and strong hair. An easy, quick, and simple way of getting all its benefits is by adding two tablespoons of chia seeds to a glass of water or to your protein shakes.

FOOD #10: COCOA POWDER

Eating healthy doesn't have to be boring. What I am about to tell you will make chocolate lovers so happy! Like all chocolate, cocoa powder comes from the cocoa bean. But it is different from the processed and unhealthy chocolate that you find in stores. This one is kept in its natural and healthy state.

Its delicious and sugarless chocolate flavor is filled with nutrients, especially magnesium (which women crave during their menstrual cycle). It is also rich in antioxidants; it contains four times the amount of antioxidants as found in green tea. You thought oolong was healthy? Try cocoa powder!

FOOD #11: APPLE CIDER VINEGAR

Apple cider vinegar is such a dream. It reduces your appetite by increasing the sensation of being full. It provides a healthy blood sugar level and suppresses all sugar cravings. More importantly, apple cider vinegar has been shown to increase insulin sensitivity, and decrease the body's ability to store fat, making it easier to melt it away.

FOOD #12: ACAI BERRY

This berry comes from the acai tree found in Central and South America. Don't be fooled by its size, its nutritional profile is huge. It is filled with antioxidants, and it has been shown to increase energy levels, digestion, immune function, and mental focus, because it is filled with nutrients that suppress appetite and cravings, helping you feel satisfied.

FOOD #13: FLAXSEED

Flaxseed has been a great ally to weight loss for many years. The plant comes from a region called Fertile Crescent, located between the Mediterranean Sea and India. Flaxseed has anti-inflammatory and antioxidant properties. Its seeds have detoxifying and anti-allergic effects and they may help prevent cancer, arthritis, as well as relieve menopausal symptoms. Flaxseed is high in dietary fiber, which helps to regulate blood pressure and blood glucose levels.

FOOD #14: TURMERIC

Studies have shown that turmeric increases the flow of bile in the stomach which helps to break down fat. Taking just one teaspoon of turmeric before each meal can help your digestion break down the fat that causes you to gain weight. In studies on mice, it was found that turmeric was an actual fat suppressant. Mice that were given turmeric gained less weight than mice on the same diet excepting the turmeric.

Another way turmeric aids in weight loss is by fighting insulin resistance and controlling sugar levels. This not only keeps you from retaining extra fat, but lowers your chances of developing diabetes. If you already have diabetes, it helps you to control your glucose numbers.

These super foods can be found in most supermarkets. But you can also get them online, in case you don't find them in a store near you.

Chapter 7

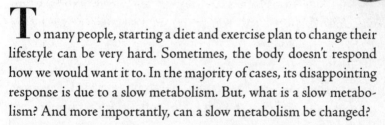

SPEED UP YOUR METABOLISM!

To many people, starting a diet and exercise plan to change their lifestyle can be very hard. Sometimes, the body doesn't respond how we would want it to. In the majority of cases, its disappointing response is due to a slow metabolism. But, what is a slow metabolism? And more importantly, can a slow metabolism be changed?

In this chapter, you will discover the reason why you can't lose weight with an out-of-control metabolism. You'll also learn how to reactivate it, almost effortlessly!

SUPERCHARGE YOUR METABOLISM!

If you feel that it is too hard to lose weight, even with all the effort; if you feel constantly tired even if you had a good night's sleep; if your muscles hurt and take too long to recover after working out, then it would be a good idea for you to pay attention to what I am going to say, because all those problems can be caused by a small, butterfly-shaped gland found under your larynx.

This gland is your thyroid. It has a *huge* effect on your body's ability to burn fat. It is the magic key to controlling your weight!

If you are one of the people who suffer from a slow thyroid, you will find it almost impossible to lose weight and burn fat around your stomach and butt. This "slow thyroid" is a condition known as "hypothyroidism," and it is out of control. More than *10 million* Americans have been diagnosed with hypothyroidism, and there are millions more waiting to be diagnosed.[3]

The thyroid gland is found in your neck and is responsible for controlling your metabolism. Its job is to segregate hormones (T3 and T4), the ones that tell our cells how fast they should burn calories to get energy. When this process fails and your thyroid is underactive, called hypothyroidism, it is shown through very unpleasant symptoms. You're always tired. Your skin and nails dry up. Your muscles hurt and recover very slowly after working out. You are always cold. You are constantly constipated. And the worst part? Your metabolism slows down, and you gain weight that is almost impossible to lose.

I understand your frustration. This condition has always been in my family. And even though I don't suffer from it, my mom and sister do, so I know how it feels.

After reading all kinds of messages from women telling me their stories, detailing their fight against hypothyroidism, and asking me how to get through this obstacle to get the sexy, slim body that they dream of, I felt the need to help them.

So I began to investigate, and I want you to know that there is hope!

3. Jeffrey R. Garber, MD, FACP, FACE, "Hypothyroidism: What Experts Suggest for Treating Low Thyroid Hormone Levels," *Empower, http://empoweryourhealth.org/magazine/vol5_issue1/Hypothyroidism_What_Experts_Suggest_for_Treating_Low_Thyroid_Hormone_Levels (accessed October 1, 2015).*

If you make some changes in your life, you can reach your weight-loss goal. These changes let you take control of the situation, get your metabolism moving, and burn fat.

Let's get started and let our thyroid know who's boss!

TAKING CHARGE

First, your diet should be high in proteins. To anybody trying to lose weight, proteins are the most important food. But when a person suffers from hypothyroidism and is trying to lose weight, it is even more important. Protein contains high thermal effects because a lot of energy is needed to decompose and digest it. This energy, of course, requires the use of calories. So, when you follow a high protein diet, your body is forced to burn the calories, which helps you lose weight.

Eat smaller portions, more often. Since hypothyroidism is linked to insulin resistance, it is important to avoid losing control of your blood sugar levels. When you eat a big meal, you will feel a massive release of insulin, which will cause those calories to store as fat. So, instead of eating three big meals, eat more often, but in smaller quantities. This will keep your sugar level under control, while you constantly feed your body with nutrients.

Avoid simple sugar. This also has to do with insulin. Consuming simple carbohydrates (such as corn, cakes, white flours, pasta, and sugary cereals) generates a release of insulin into the body because these foods digest quickly and are used as short-term energy. Since we want to keep the insulin levels stable, we should avoid these foods.

Focus on complex carbohydrates. When you suffer from hypothyroidism, complex carbohydrates are your best allies. They contain a huge source of energy. But, since the energy is released slowly, it doesn't affect your insulin levels the way that simple carbohydrates do. A good way to include these carbohydrates into your diet is by including fruits and all kinds of colorful vegetables.

The super vegetables and fresh fruits are highly recommended. But pay attention, because some vegetables from the cabbage family and some fruits should be eaten in very small quantities since they block the iodine use and absorption, which makes the thyroid gland activity stop and worsens your condition. These foods include Brussels sprouts, cauliflower, kale, spinach, mustard leaves, swede, turnip, millet, strawberries, peaches, peanuts, horse radish, and soy beans. But this doesn't mean that you should never eat them; just remember to cook them first, to destroy the goitrogens.

I don't recommend consuming soy foods, such as tofu, milk, and protein bars, since soy prevents the cell receptors from functioning and interrupts and disrupts the hormonal endocrine system.

Eat fats! Good fats, such as olive oil, avocados, flaxseeds, fish, and nuts, can do miracles since your body needs them to produce more hormones.

Consume minerals to have a "healthy thyroid." There are certain essential minerals for the proper functioning of the thyroid. When one is missing, the metabolism slows down and burns fewer calories. To avoid this, you need to maintain the mineral levels in the body. The thyroid needs iodine to produce hormones. A good source of iodine is found in seafood, sea vegetables, and fruits such as strawberries and blueberries. Zinc and selenium are other minerals that help the T3 levels stay leveled. Selenium is found in lamb, fish, eggs, seafood, and onions, for a few examples. To get zinc, eat nuts, oysters, meats, pumpkin seeds, and wheat germ.

Avoid coffee! Caffeine (plus the added sugar) creates unnecessary stress on your adrenal glands, which work in synergy with the thyroid. When you develop adrenal gland fatigue, due to caffeine, you make hypothyroidism worse.

Avoid alcohol! This one's obvious! Alcohol dehydrates you and depletes you of mineral sources. It also alters your ability to think clearly, makes you hungry, especially for unhealthy foods, and in general, and adds to your daily caloric count—especially if you're drinking mixed drinks or beer. As you can see, the cumulative effect of alcohol will ruin your metabolism.

Get moving! A low-impact exercise improves health and joint movement. It also burns calories and helps you to lose weight because you're making sure that the consumed carbohydrates get used as energy and not stored as fat.

It is not a coincidence that these changes help people feel "good" and look even better, whether or not they suffer from hypothyroidism. Having good eating habits makes your body work at its best.

When you include these changes into your life, your body doesn't have another option but to respond. Provide it with a constant flow of nutrients and avoid processed foods. You will be amazed at how fast your metabolism improves and how quickly you begin to lose weight!

So make these changes whenever possible, and finally feel how the frustration and slow metabolism start to become a thing from the past. I know this will make a huge difference in your life!

METABOLISM AT FULL SPEED!

There is a vital rule to losing weight: keep your metabolism at full speed. If it slows down, you gain weight.

How do we do this? Easy. As I mentioned before, make sure you eat more than three meals a day. Now, remember that this is not about only eating, but eating healthily, and consuming the proper foods for your body. Let's talk about this in more detail.

First, start your day with a good breakfast. Since you have been fasting for so many hours during the night, while resting, your first meal will activate your body and give it the first impulse that it needs to start working. Similar to motivating yourself to start the day, you have to also motivate your metabolism.

For this first meal, don't eat any refined carbohydrates, because these can cause you to lack energy by midmorning. Instead of eating a doughnut for breakfast, opt to eat good quality carbohydrates instead!

Be creative! Proteins, good fats, and good, complex carbohydrates in the morning will give you much more energy to start the day. At the same time, a complete meal will start your metabolism at full speed, making you burn fat.

Maybe a slice of turkey breast with avocado on a piece of whole wheat bread sounds appealing. Or how about some oatmeal with a little fruit? It won't increase your sugar levels, so you won't feel tired by midmorning, and since your body digests these kinds of breakfasts more slowly, they will help you feel full for longer.

Another tip, which is a little older and which we don't hear often enough, is to drink a lot of water. Water hydrates, and when you are hydrated, your health improves. Don't forget to drink your eight glasses of water a day! You will feel satisfied and your metabolism will continue to move. If you get tired of only drinking water, don't worry. As I mentioned in a previous chapter, green tea is an excellent substitute, due to the ECGC plant, that helps to burn fat faster.

If you like spicy food, you are in luck, because a tablespoon of hot chilies can accelerate your metabolism, up to 23%! So add it to your salads and fresh salsas.

Lastly, don't forget the vegetables. Dark leafy vegetables such as spinach or Chinese cabbage are high in iron, and are very important for women, especially during their period.

And how about some exercise? You do understand how important this is, right? Exercise is essential to accelerating your metabolism and keeping your body strong and healthy. And the best part is that you don't have to spend hours in a gym; instead, do interval training. Don't spend an hour running the same speed on the treadmill, but run short and intense cycles. For example, you could spend twenty minutes on the treadmill doing an interval routine, walking for one minute, then running for one minute, until you complete twenty minutes. This type of routine will help you to accelerate your metabolism and fat loss.

After all that activity, don't forget to get your rest! Sleeping is so good—and so important! Sleep at least six to eight hours every night. If you don't sleep enough, your leptin and ghrelin levels will get unbalanced. You need them to be balanced and happy because they regulate the appetite and energy. The last thing you need is your body complaining at ten o'clock in the evening that you need to eat the whole fridge. Sometimes when your body is telling you it's hungry, what it really means is that it's sleepy!

Finally, please, don't try to accelerate your metabolism by drinking coffee or any other caffeinated drink. Even if these drinks give you energy, it is only of a temporary kind. In less than an hour, I guarantee that you will be tired again. Also, they don't do anything to your metabolism and they cause health problems.

Accelerating your metabolism in a healthy way will help you burn pounds quicker and soon enough you will be able to wear those jeans—or whatever other sexy clothing item is hanging in your closet!

7 METABOLISM-BOOSTING FOODS

If you have ever read my blog, you know that I don't recommend diets. I want to motivate you to lose weight by adopting a new lifestyle that includes eating well and doing exercises.

One of the healthiest ways of losing weight is simply burning fat. You do this by keeping your metabolism moving. When you take care of your metabolism, you are not only helping yourself to burn fat, but you also have more energy. You can't sit around and get depressed when your metabolism is telling you to move, move, move!

Today I want to talk about seven foods that are excellent for accelerating your metabolism. Eating these foods will help you burn all those extra calories and will make you lose weight a lot faster; they will also help you to avoid gaining those pounds back!

Here are my seven favorite foods:

1. Artichoke: This vegetable can be prepared by steaming it with a little oil. By only eating a medium size artichoke, you will get some protein and fiber. It also has the perfect amount of calories to increase your metabolism and burn fat.

2. Vinegar: It not only helps you increase your metabolism, but also can increase your insulin sensibility and delay your sugar level increment. Drink a glass of water with one or two tablespoons of vinegar before eating, and you will push your metabolism and at the same time suppress your appetite.

3. Seaweed: Not only is seaweed delicious, but it also helps you move your metabolism. It is often used in sushi, but can also be used in salads, sautés, shakes, soups, or even on fish to give it more flavor. A lot of people like to make tea with kombu algae. There are different kinds of algae, but most of them are highly rich in minerals and vitamins.

4. Oolong tea: Forget the coffee and drink some tea instead! It will accelerate your metabolism without the harmful side effects of coffee.

5. Cinnamon. Eat a tablespoon of cinnamon twenty minutes before eating, and your metabolism will kick into

high gear. Studies show that cinnamon can lower blood sugar levels and stabilize your glucose levels. You can drink a tablespoon of cinnamon in hot water or add it to your foods, such as potatoes or oatmeal, to give them more flavor.

6. Cayenne pepper: Spicy food is not only delicious, it also helps you to feel satisfied with less food. Cayenne pepper also contains capsaicin, which helps you to burn calories for at least twenty or thirty minutes after consumption.

7. Ginger: This little root is another spice that will make your metabolism jump, often up to 20% or more, while also helping out your digestion. A little minced ginger adds a flavorful kick to your stir-fry, and many people also enjoy adding it to their shakes.

Chapter 8

DARE TO USE THESE MENTAL TRICKS!

You may think that I have gone crazy, but there are many ways to cheat your body and your mind that will help you out in incredible ways. Trust me; I have become my own cheater! Here is a small list of how you can train your body to do more of what you like, and less of what you don't like:

1. DRINK A GLASS OF WATER BEFORE EATING.

During my transformation, I used this trick before every meal. When you drink a glass of water before eating, you are cheating your body, making it think that it's satisfied.

"Why would you want to eat less than what your body needs?" you may ask. Well, that's the trick. Americans think that they need a huge portion of food to be satisfied. That's a terrible myth.

Drinking water won't keep you from eating what you need, it will keep you from eating *more* than you need.

2. USE SMALLER PLATES, INSTEAD OF BIG ONES.

I know you have heard this before, but it really works! When we use big plates, we tend to eat everything on it; and probably, eat more than what we should, without really noticing it.

However, if you eat your food on a small plate, you will have a lot less food, and once you are finished with your plate, your mind will think that you are done. It will send a signal to your brain for you to stop eating, and it will feel like the most natural thing in the world to put down your fork and get up to clear the table.

3. CHEW YOUR FOOD TWENTY-FIVE TIMES BEFORE SWALLOWING.

This tricks your stomach into thinking that you are eating more, when you are actually eating a lot less. Chewing your food twenty-five times before swallowing and putting your fork down between bites will help you fill up faster.

Why does this happen? Because when you take time to chew, it is easier for your body to digest the food, and it gives you a satiating feeling a whole lot faster.

4. BRUSH YOUR TEETH WHEN YOU FEEL LIKE EATING SWEETS!

The clean sensation in your mouth will stop you from eating sweets. While you are in the bathroom, brushing your teeth, take a look at the picture of when you were skinny. Between the fresh breath and the picture, your sugar cravings will disappear.

I think you are starting to have a better idea on how to work this new habit! Instead of being about the specific diet or exercise program that you choose, it's really all about *what's in your head*, and *how you handle* the diet or exercise program.

CHEAT MEALS

I think I have made myself very clear in this section, but, in case I didn't, I want to clarify a little more, because what you are doing to achieve a healthier life is very brave and it is not impossible. Your main focus should be that you are doing something amazing for yourself. Remember this always: with great sacrifice comes great rewards!

A great way to reward yourself after a week full of challenges is with a cheat meal. Once a week, eat whatever you want. Yes, you heard me right! Pizza? Why not? Chinese food? All yours! Ice cream and chocolate cravings? Go for it!

This is your chance to take advantage of any meal that you have been craving all week. Adding this weekly cheat meal works wonders for your metabolism and helps you reach your goals.

One and only one!

By cheating once per week, you're able to get your cravings out so you can stick to the eating plan the rest of the week without trouble. Let's say that you go out to dinner with your family, and you want to eat that plate of pasta that you love so much. You tell yourself, *I want this now, but I'll save it for my cheat meal.* It will be much easier to avoid it, knowing that you can order it on your cheat meal day.

A cheat meal will not only give you the willpower that you need during the week, but it will also give you more energy and will increase your metabolism.

One important note: always eat your cheat meal on the same day, at the same time. That way, you won't get confused about when was the last time you cheated. Choose the day that's most convenient to you.

I always liked to have my cheat meal on Sunday afternoons. I didn't want it too late in the evening because I didn't want the unhealthy food I was eating to sit in my system overnight.

By loading up in the afternoon, I found that my workouts the next day were amazing! Whatever extra calories I took in during the meal were easily burned off during my workout because I had the extra energy to really push myself in the gym.

You have already done the hardest thing: *you made the decision to change your life!* So why not reward yourself occasionally?

Chapter 9

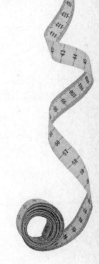

HOW DO YOU GET STARTED?

I know you are extremely excited to change your life, change your body, and improve your health. You are tired of looking at "you" in the mirror—and then feeling a mad urge to break the mirror into little pieces. You are ready to look into the mirror and think, *Wow! Is that me? I look great!*

It's time to change! *But how should you get started?*

Once you have made the decision to take control of your life, there are some things that you need to do before going to the gym, or beginning your new food plan. Even if this sounds crazy, it is necessary.

You need to change some things in your house, or they'll become an obstacle when you're trying to lose weight.

And yes, I'm talking about the kitchen.

That place where you spend hours a day, making delicious meals and putting away groceries that, frankly, shouldn't even exist. So go to your kitchen, stand in the middle, and look around. You will see all the food that you have been eating and that you now know are not healthy.

So, what do you do?

JUNK FOOD GOES IN THE TRASH!

During the first stages of losing weight, you should get rid of all obstacles that can ruin your resolve. Eventually, once you have established a mind-set and once eating healthy has become a habit, you will be able to resist the temptation more easily. But before that happens, you need to avoid anything that may cause you to fail.

You see, the biggest temptations won't take place when you're out and about, busy at work, or running errands. The things that are really going to test you are sitting right in your very home—in your cabinets, in your pantry, and in your fridge.

With junk food littering your kitchen, all it takes is one moment of weakness to give in and set yourself back. One moment to lose the momentum we're so desperately after. We just aren't willing to take that risk! That's why the next step on your weight-loss journey is to find these unhealthy temptations hiding in your kitchen—and throw them away!

That's right, get rid of them! I want you to inspect all the food in your kitchen, going over each and every box and bag with the detail of a police detective. And just think about whether it's going to help you or hinder you.

Throw out anything you know you should not be eating. Anything that you know is going to end up around your butt and thighs, trash it. All the cereals, sugary drinks, white bread, pasta, chips, sodas, candy, desserts, doughnuts, pastries, toss it right into the garbage.

Now I know this might seem a bit silly to you, but this step is so important. It allows your subconscious to process the fact that you're taking this seriously. After all, it's one thing to say you're going to do something, but to actually see it being done takes things to a different level.

So as you throw all of these unhealthy foods away, not only are you tossing out temptation, but you're also saying goodbye to the old you.

As you toss out those fattening foods and sugary soft drinks, you're also saying goodbye to all of the bad habits that have kept you from your goals, all of the toxic pounds that have been weighing you down.

If you want to make this step even more effective, get your family involved in it. You have already informed them of your goals as part of building your support structure, so why not have them help to directly toss out the junk?

Now hear me out on this, because this part can be tricky, especially with your children. Changing your eating habits is a great opportunity for you to set an example for them and to educate them on how important it is to be healthy, to consciously see what they should and should not be eating.

Involving them gives you the chance to explain what it is you're doing. They need to know the reasons behind the changes. We don't want them to think that mommy or daddy have just gone crazy and started throwing all the food away! Explain that you're not interested in wasting food; you're interested in buying better food in the future. Explain to them what is going on and how you're trying to become happier and healthier.

Trust me, I have kids, and I know how hard it is to get them to part with their favorite chips or gummies. I want to make it clear to you, and you need to make this clear to them; this isn't about depriving them of their favorite treats! Kids are supposed to be kids and can get away with enjoying these treats.

But treats are exactly that—*treats*! You don't take them to the zoo every day, that's a treat. You don't let them buy a new outfit every day, that's a treat. Treats are to be enjoyed on rare occasions. Let them have them in school, or if you're out shopping. But there is no reason to have all this unhealthy food laying around the house; all that does is instill bad habits in them. And you know from personal experience how hard it is to break those habits!

So make it easy on your kids, and throw that junk away! Your entire family will be better off because of it.

GROCERY SHOPPING SECRETS

Many health lovers will tell you that abs are made in the kitchen.

They make these types of comments to emphasize the importance of a well-balanced diet. It doesn't matter how much you work out in a gym; if you are not eating correctly, you are not going to see the results that you want.

But, as much as I agree with that saying, it is wrong, because many people are doomed to fail before they even step into their kitchen! Why?

Because they sabotage their efforts when they go to the supermarket! When they go grocery shopping, they make mistakes that make it almost impossible to reach their goal.

I am going to clear up some common mistakes and show you what you can do next time you go shopping!

SLIMMING SECRET #1: NEVER GO TO THE SUPERMARKET HUNGRY!

One of the biggest mistakes that you can make is to go grocery shopping on an empty stomach. When you are hungry, your decision-making ability is affected. Try to go early in the day, when you are really awake and alert. This will help you make the best decisions.

SLIMMING SECRET #2: IF IT'S NOT ON THE LIST, DON'T BUY IT!

The best way to avoid buying unhealthy foods is by making a list and sticking to it! If it is written on the list, it goes in the cart; if it's not, then it stays in the supermarket. This simple rule will save you a lot of regret.

SLIMMING SECRET #3: DO YOUR SHOPPING FROM THE OUTSIDE TO THE INSIDE.

Most supermarkets are designed in a way that the healthy foods are on the outer or side shelves, so that they can easily be restocked. And guess what—they need to be restocked because they're *fresh* and *healthy*. That is where we usually find the fruits, vegetables, fish, and meat. These are essential ingredients to a balanced meal plan.

Make it a habit to go into the supermarket and grab the essentials first from the outer aisles. Then, if there is something on the list that you need to get, you can stroll down the inner aisles (where the junk food is).

SLIMMING SECRET #4: IF YOU CAN'T PRONOUNCE IT, DON'T BUY IT!

Many times, you ask yourself if you should be eating a specific food. Well, follow this simple rule and you'll never be confused again: Only buy foods that you can pronounce.

Most probably, the one ingredient that you can't pronounce will be an artificial or additive ingredient that is not good for your health.

To prove my theory, let's look at two example foods:

Food #1:

Ingredients: *chicken breast.*

Food #2:

Ingredients: *sugar, unbleached enriched flour (wheat flour, niacin, reduced iron, thiamine mononitrate {vitamin B1}, riboflavin {vitamin B2}, folic acid), palm and/or canola oil, cocoa (processed with alkali), high fructose corn syrup, cornstarch, leavening (baking soda and/or calcium phosphate), salt, soy lecithin, vanillin – an artificial flavor, chocolate. Contains wheat, soy.*

It is easy to see which one of these ingredients is healthier, right? (The second one is the ingredients for an Oreo cookie, in case you are wondering.)

If you follow these simple tips when you go grocery shopping, you will be able to avoid many mistakes that sabotage your efforts to lose weight.

Here is some advice that has worked wonderfully for me: go grocery shopping right after the gym, when you are still all sweaty (make sure to eat a small snack). Your mind will still be in "healthy" mode. When you stroll down the aisles, you will be choosing wisely because you are conscious of the work you have done at the gym—and you don't want it to go to waste.

Instead of thinking, *Wow, that cheesecake looks amazing…let's get it!* your thought process will be more like, *Do I want a cheesecake after dinner? Of course! But there is no way I'm burning those calories off.*

People are often very adamant about whether you "need" or "don't need" to count calories. Some say that it is absolutely necessary, while others say that it is a waste of time. This is my opinion: read the labels. Read the calories, sodium, carbohydrates, sugars, everything. Read all the ingredients in the back of the label.

This exercise is not to count the amount of calories or carbohydrates; instead, this is to understand completely what you are putting in your mouth. Remember, if you have no idea how to pronounce an ingredient, don't buy it! Succumbing to temptation when grocery shopping is normal; that happens to everyone. The trick is to be strong!

Do you know the difference between a person who is in shape and a person who is not? One has willpower, the other doesn't.

You can do it! This is your first step. Afterward, you'll be thinking, *That wasn't so hard!*

Chapter 10

LET'S BEGIN: START YOUR BODY TRANSFORMATION NOW!

Kick-start your new figure!

This is so exciting! You are well on your way to a new life. There's no turning back, we are in it together, and we will come out victorious from this challenge.

Now that we understand the process and the things that we need to change, it is time to show you how to transform your body. For that, I have designed a 5-day plan that I know you've been waiting for. This will give you the push that your body needs to be ready for and to start your new lifestyle, so let's see it!

WELCOME TO THE KICK-START OF THE NEW YOU!

I am so excited that you have decided to join me in this journey. Congratulate yourself. Feel proud, because you have made the best choice.

Now, over the next 5 short days, I'm going to help you turn your dreams into reality. In just 5 short days, we're going to undo literally years of bad habits. Any mistakes you've made in the past simply do not matter. If you've tried diets and failed, it's no big deal. If you've slacked off on the exercise, it's not a problem. If you've eaten foods you know you shouldn't have eaten, forget about it! None of that matters anymore.

We're wiping the slate clean and giving you the fresh start you deserve. All I ask is that you give me your best effort for these 5 short days. If you can promise me that, then I promise to help you take control of your health, your body...and your life!

I know how hard it can be to get started. I've been where you've been, desperately wanting to change, but not knowing how to take that first step. But once I figured it out, I was able to drop 55 pounds in 90 days. And in this 5-day program, I'm going to put you on the right path to reaching your goals, whatever they may be.

We're going to free your body from the toxins that have been slowing down your metabolism. We're going to eliminate all that stored "junk" that's been causing you to hold onto those stubborn pounds, so that, in just 5 short days from now, your body is in the perfect condition to start melting fat, easier than you ever thought possible.

You're no longer weighed down by the chemicals and toxins of processed food. You're no longer reliant on sugar and caffeine to get you through the day. Instead, your body gets all the energy it needs from a much greater source...*delicious, nutritious, natural foods!*

These foods provide you with clean energy throughout your entire day, without the "crashes" you're used to. By eating these foods, you give your body the break it desperately craves. You give it the "jump start" it needs to start melting fat!

You see, each day, we're constantly stuffing our bodies full of toxins.

They're in the food we eat (especially processed food), the air we breathe, and the chemicals we clean with. It's no wonder that, over time, our bodies become overloaded. These toxins are very dangerous to our health.

So in order to keep us safe, to protect us from getting sick or even dying, our bodies store these toxins away. And one of the places it prefers to store them is in our fat cells! That's why the more toxic you are...the more likely you are to store excess body fat!

Since your body has to dedicate so much energy to keeping these toxins contained, your metabolism comes to a screeching halt. But when you remove those toxins from your system, your body no longer has to spend all its resources fighting them off.

When you start providing your body with high levels of nutrients, like the fruit and vegetables we're going to be eating, suddenly it has energy to spare. And it's able to use that energy to improve itself.

You're able to think more clearly, your circulation improves; your skin develops that youthful glow again. You look and feel healthy, because without these toxins weighing you down, you *are* healthy! And you will have the healthy fat-burning metabolism to go along with it!

That's exactly what this 5-day program is designed to do. It's going to give your body a "jump start" back to health. That being said, this program is not intended for long-term use. It's only designed to be used for 5 days.

And this jump start program will put you in the perfect position to get the greatest results. So before we move onto the meat of the program, let me give you two quick tips.

First, you aren't going to want to lift weights during this program…or do any strenuous exercise. Your body is going to be under enough stress from dealing with built-up toxins. You don't want to be adding to this stress.

However, you should still be active! You want to keep your blood pumping to help eliminate these toxins from your system. So you should do thirty to forty minutes of low intensity exercise each day during this program, such as walking, biking, yoga, etc. As long as it's at a comfortable pace, it doesn't matter what exactly it is. The important thing is to keep that blood flowing.

Second, in order to help speed up the "detoxification process," we're going to be taking "detox showers." Here's how it works: After you take your regular shower, before you get out, I want you to turn the water as hot as you can stand (without getting burned) for sixty seconds. Then, turn it as cold as you can stand for another minute. Repeat this process three times. It will increase the circulation to your skin and open your pores, allowing the toxins to pass through. You'll find that this helps cut out a lot of the "side effects" people commonly report when detoxifying, such as headaches. It also speeds up the process, getting you greater results in less time.

And as long as you understand everything so far, we're ready to move on with the rest of the "jump start" program.

So get excited, because we're about to create the "new you"!

11 IMPORTANT RULES THAT GUARANTEE GREAT RESULTS!

1. Please, do *not* skip any meals. This plan was carefully designed and should be followed as written in order to deliver the greatest results.

2. It is important to eat every three hours from the moment you wake up to when you go to sleep, in order to keep your metabolism burning at full speed.

3. If you do not find the listed ingredients, use your creativity and replace them with similar items that are in season.

4. It is important to drink the recommended amounts of water with each meal.

5. If you find yourself hungry between meals, snack on some salt-free almonds.

6. To speed up the process, be sure to stay active. I recommend 30–40 minutes of low-intensity cardio each day.

7. To detoxify you must *not* chew gum, consume dairy, or eat sweets. You also need to stay away from drinking alcohol or coffee…both of which dehydrate you. The *only* things you should be drinking are water or tea (green, red, detox, black, oolong, etc.) during and between your meals. For best results, you can add skinny tea & colon tea from www.IMDetoxTea.com.

8. You can eat all the green vegetables or lettuce you want. These foods are high in fiber, yet incredibly low in calories. This makes them the perfect food to fill up on guilt-free.

9. Do not add any artificial seasonings or condiments to your food. To keep it simple, we're going to stick to salt and pepper so we don't interfere with the detoxification process.

10. When you follow this "jump start" diet correctly, not only will you feel rejuvenated and filled with energy, but your body will be in the perfect condition to start easily dropping pounds!

11. Be positive and *always* smile. Remember, you're looking better, feeling better, and becoming better every day. You have many reasons to be happy!

(If you suffer from a particular medical condition, it is important to check with your doctor before you start any diet. Remember that if you suffer from hypothyroidism, you can replace some of the green vegetables for others of the same category.)

SHOPPING LIST

Fruits:

+ Lemon or lime
+ Green apple
+ Banana
+ Strawberry
+ Blueberry

Vegetables:

+ Spinach
+ Celery
+ Ginger
+ Lettuce
+ Cilantro/coriander
+ Asparagus
+ Broccoli

Legumes:

+ Avocado
+ Carrot
+ Onion
+ Artichoke

Grains:

+ Chickpeas
+ Lentils

Whole wheat products:

+ Quinoa

Dressings:

+ Honey
+ Olive oil

- Balsamic vinegar
- Liquid aminos (or low-sodium soy sauce)
- Rice vinegar
- Sesame oil

Others:

- Tofu
- Green tea or herbal tea (decaffeinated)
- Sea salt
- Pepper

Seeds:

- Chia seeds or Flaxseed
- Pumpkin seeds
- Almonds
- Cranberries or raisins

MENU TO JUMP-START YOUR NEW BODY

Here's your 5-day detox shortcut to a slim, healthy body!

DAY #1

Breakfast:

Juice: 1 green apple
1 bunch of spinach
2 celery stalks
1 thumb-size piece of ginger
1 banana
1 Tbsp. chia seeds (or 1 Tbsp. flaxseed)
½ cup green tea

Preparation: Add all the vegetables to the blender and add a ½ cup water or green tea, then add the chia seeds and blend for 60 seconds; it's now ready to drink!

Beverage: 1 cup hot water with ½ squeezed lemon

Snack #1:

> ¼ cup mixture of pumpkin seeds, almonds, and Craisins
>
> ½ green apple

Beverage: 16 oz. of water (or 2 big glasses) and 1 cup green tea or detox tea, decaffeinated and flavorless

Lunch:

Spinach Salad

> 3 cups spinach
>
> ½ block of tofu
>
> ¼ cup almonds
>
> 1 cup raw broccoli
>
> ½ small avocado

Dressing:

> 1 Tbsp. liquid aminos (or low-sodium soy sauce)
>
> 3 Tbsp. sesame oil
>
> 2 Tbsp. rice vinegar

Preparation: Cut the tofu into medium size cubes, season with sea salt and pepper. On a hot pan, lightly coat with non-stick coconut oil spray; add the tofu. Cook for 8 to 10 minutes until golden. Remove from heat. Combine the rest of the ingredients, and toss with dressing.

Snack #2:

> ¼ cup mixture of pumpkin seeds, almonds, and Craisins
>
> ½ green apple

Beverage: 16 oz. of water (or 2 big glasses) and 1 cup green tea or detox tea, decaffeinated and flavorless

Dinner:

Artichoke Soup

> 3 cups water
>
> ½ cup chopped carrots
>
> ½ onion, chopped
>
> 2 celery stalks, chopped
>
> 1 cup artichokes (or small can)*

Preparation: In a saucepan, add the carrots, celery stalks, and onions; cook for 20 minutes. Remove the liquid and add the artichokes, cook with the rest of the ingredients for 5 minutes. Carefully mix all the ingredients in a blender. Enjoy!

*Natural artichokes take a bit longer to cook (about an hour). If you can't find it, you can replace it with any other vegetable in season.

Beverage: 8 oz. of water (or a small glass)

DAY #2

Breakfast:

Juice: 1 green apple

> 1 bunch of spinach
>
> 2 celery stalks
>
> 1 thumb-size piece of ginger
>
> 1 banana
>
> 1 Tbsp. chia seeds (or 1 Tbsp. flaxseed)
>
> ½ cup green tea

Preparation: Add all the vegetables to the blender and add a ½ cup water or green tea, then add the chia seeds and blend for 60 seconds; it's now ready to drink.

Beverage: 1 cup hot water with ½ squeezed lemon

Snack #1:

> ¼ cup mixture of pumpkin seeds, almonds, and Craisins
>
> ½ green apple

Beverage: 16 oz. of water (or 2 big glasses) and 1 cup green tea or detox tea, decaffeinated and flavorless

Lunch:

Lentil salad

> 2 cups spinach
>
> ½ cup lentils, raw
>
> 1 lime, juiced
>
> ½ white onion, chopped
>
> 1 celery stalk, diced
>
> ½ small carrot, grated
>
> ½ parsley, minced
>
> 2 Tbsp. olive oil
>
> Sea salt and pepper

Preparation: Add lentils to a saucepan and cover them with water by 2 inches. Cover the pan with a tight fitting lid and bring to a boil over medium-high heat, about 10 minutes. Uncover, reduce the heat to medium low, and simmer, stirring occasionally, for 15 minutes. Add 1 teaspoon of sea salt, stir to combine, and continue to simmer until the lentils are just tender, about 10 to 12 minutes more. Remove from heat and drain. In a large bowl, mix all the ingredients and add lime juice, olive oil, sea salt, and pepper. Toss salad to coat with dressing.

Snack #2:

> ¼ cup mixture of pumpkin seeds, almonds, and Craisins
>
> ½ green apple

Beverage: 16 oz. of water (or 2 big glasses) and 1 cup green tea or detox tea, decaffeinated and flavorless

Dinner:

Ginger and Carrot Soup

> 3 carrots, quartered
>
> 1 tsp. of grated ginger
>
> 2 cups water
>
> ⅓ cup almond milk
>
> 1 chopped onion
>
> Sea salt and pepper to taste

Preparation: Add all the ingredients in a saucepan and cook them on medium heat for 25 minutes. Carefully mix all the ingredients in the blender. Enjoy!

Beverage: 8 oz. of water (or a small glass)

DAY #3

Breakfast:

Juice: 1 green apple

> 1 bunch of spinach
>
> 2 celery stalks
>
> 1 thumb-size piece of ginger
>
> 1 banana
>
> 1 Tbsp. chia seeds (or 1 Tbsp. flaxseed)
>
> ½ cup green tea

Preparation: Add all the vegetables to the blender and add a ½ cup water or green tea, then add the chia seeds and blend for 60 seconds; it's now ready to drink.

Beverage: 1 cup hot water with ½ squeezed lemon

Snack #1:

> ¼ cup mixture of pumpkin seeds, almonds, and Craisins
>
> ½ green apple

Beverage: 16 oz. of water (or 2 big glasses) and 1 cup green tea or detox tea, decaffeinated and flavorless

Lunch:

Chickpea Salad

> 2 cups spinach
>
> ½ cup canned chickpeas (low-sodium)
>
> 1 bunch fresh parsley, finely chopped
>
> 2 Tbsp. red onion
>
> 1 celery stalk
>
> 2 limes, juiced
>
> 1 Tbsp. olive oil
>
> Sea salt and pepper

Preparation: Combine all the ingredients in a medium size mixing bowl.

Beverage: 1 cup green or red tea, decaffeinated and flavorless

Snack #2:

> ¼ cup mixture of pumpkin seeds, almonds, and Craisins
>
> ½ green apple

Beverage: 16 oz. of water (or 2 big glasses) and 1 cup green tea or detox tea, decaffeinated and flavorless

Dinner:

Spinach Soup

> 2 cups water
> ½ cup chopped onion
> 3 cups spinach
> ½ cup chopped carrot
> 1 stalk of celery
> Sea salt and pepper to taste

Preparation: Add all the ingredients to a saucepan and cook them for 25 minutes at medium heat. Carefully blend all the ingredients. Enjoy!

Beverage: 8 oz. of water (or a small glass)

DAY #4

Breakfast:

Juice:　1 green apple
> 1 bunch of spinach
> 2 celery stalks
> 1 thumb-size piece of ginger
> 1 banana
> 1 Tbsp. chia seeds (or 1 Tbsp. flaxseed)
> ½ cup green tea

Preparation: Add all the vegetables to the blender and add a ½ cup water or green tea, then add the chia seeds and blend for 60 seconds; it's now ready to drink.

Beverage: 1 cup hot water with ½ squeezed lemon

Snack #1:

> ¼ cup mixture of pumpkin seeds, almonds, and Craisins
>
> ½ green apple

Beverage: 16 oz. of water (or 2 big glasses) and 1 cup green tea or detox tea, decaffeinated and flavorless

Lunch:

Berry Salad

> 2 cups spinach, raw
>
> ½ cup blueberries, sliced
>
> ½ cup strawberries, sliced
>
> ½ block of tofu
>
> ⅓ cup walnuts

Preparation: In a heated pan, sauté tofu and transfer to a plate. Wash berries thoroughly, slice, and serve with tofu and spinach. Mix and toss salad to coat with dressing.

Strawberry Vinaigrette

> 5 strawberries
>
> 1 Tbsp. Balsamic vinegar
>
> 3 Tbsp. olive oil
>
> Sea salt and pepper

Preparation: Mix all the ingredients in a blender and serve.

Snack #2:

> ¼ cup mixture of pumpkin seeds, almonds, and Craisins
>
> ½ green apple

Beverage: 16 oz. of water (or 2 big glasses) and 1 cup green tea or detox tea, decaffeinated and flavorless

Dinner:

Asparagus Soup

> 3 cups water
>
> 10 green asparagus
>
> ½ cup chopped onion
>
> ½ cup diced carrot
>
> 1 stalk of celery, diced
>
> Sea salt and pepper to taste

Preparation: Add all the ingredients in a saucepan and cook them at a medium heat for 25 minutes. Carefully blend them. Enjoy!

*Note: If you are not able to find asparagus you can replace them with any other green vegetable in season.

Beverage: 8 oz. of water (or a small glass)

DAY #5

Breakfast:

Juice: 1 green apple

> 1 bunch of spinach
>
> 2 celery stalks
>
> 1 thumb-size piece of ginger
>
> 1 banana
>
> 1 Tbsp. chia seeds (or 1 Tbsp. flaxseed)
>
> ½ cup green tea

Preparation: Add all the vegetables to the blender and add a ½ cup water or green tea, then add the chia seeds and blend for 60 seconds; it's now ready to drink.

Beverage: 1 cup hot water with ½ squeezed lemon

Snack #1:

    ¼ cup mixture of pumpkin seeds, almonds, and Craisins

    ½ green apple

Beverage: 16 oz. of water (or 2 big glasses) and 1 cup green tea or detox tea, decaffeinated and flavorless

Lunch:

Quinoa Salad

    2 cups spinach, raw

    ½ cup uncooked quinoa (can be replaced with brown rice)

    1 bunch fresh mint leaves, minced

    1 celery stalk, diced

    ½ cup carrot, grated

    1 bunch fresh parsley

    2 limes, juiced

    10 almonds

    1 tbsp. olive oil

    Sea salt and pepper to taste

Preparation: Combine all the ingredients in a medium size mixing bowl.

How to cook the Quinoa (double the recipe if you want leftovers):

1. To wash the quinoa, stir it with your hand and drain the clear water using a fine mesh strainer.

2. Put the quinoa into a saucepan with 1 cup water and ¼ Tbsp. salt, and bring to a boil.

3. Cook it for 15 minutes at a low temperature.

4. Before removing from the heat, add the juice of one lemon.

5. Remove it from the heat and let it sit for 5 minutes with the lid on.

6. Uncover the saucepan and stir it with a fork.

Snack #2:

> ¼ cup mixture of pumpkin seeds, almonds, and Craisins
>
> ½ green apple

Beverage: 16 oz. of water (or 2 big glasses) and 1 cup green tea or detox tea, decaffeinated and flavorless

Dinner:

Broccoli Soup

> ½ lb. of broccoli
>
> 2 cups water
>
> 1 onion, chopped
>
> 1 carrot, quartered
>
> 1 celery stalk, chunked

Preparation: Add all the ingredients in a saucepan and cook them at a medium heat for 25 minutes. Carefully blend them all together. Enjoy!

Beverage: 8 oz. of water (or a small glass)

CONGRATULATIONS!

You've successfully completed your New Body Jump Start program! You should feel proud of yourself; you made it to the end! Now, the 5 toughest days of your entire weight-loss journey are behind you forever! It only gets easier from here. You've laid the foundation and given your body the break it desperately needed. You've supplied your body with nutrients which helped eliminate harmful, metabolism-slowing toxins from your system. You may already find that you have more energy than before. But now isn't the time to stop. Now that you have your mind and body on the same page, the stage is set for quick and easy weight loss. You can finally lose all your unwanted pounds and inches...more easily than ever before!

Chapter 11

THE FORMULA TO KICK-START THE NEW YOU

Here is where the 21-day challenge that will change your life starts!

You are about to make a huge change in your life! You have detoxified your body; you have gotten rid of all the impurities and excess that didn't let you move forward in your journey of becoming healthier and happier. Now, in this chapter, I encourage you to take the leap that will change your life. We are talking about 21 days in which you are going to make, not only a physical change, but also a mental change, because these 21 days will give you the strength and conviction to move forward.

Let me explain why.

Did you know that it takes 21 days for your brain to adopt a new habit? That's right. It is scientifically proven that when we overcome the 21-day psychological boundary of letting go of old habits, or adapting to a new life situation, routine, activity, or system, we can actually say that we have *overcome* the trial.

In these 21 days, the brain takes the information and makes it its own. If we eat in a conscious, healthy, and disciplined way for 21 days, without interruptions, we can actually say that our eating habits have changed.

Doesn't this excite you? It excites me! I know how the whole "before and after" feels. I know, firsthand, how it feels when you look in the mirror and you are not happy with what you see; when you can dream of wearing an amazing dress, but know that it is impossible with the figure you have; when you try to jump, run, and play with your kids, and your body simply doesn't respond... and worst, when your health is damaged by the extra pounds, the cholesterol, or blood sugar. That's when you painfully realize, *I have no control over my life.*

Believe me; I know what it's like to be there.

That's why, in this chapter, I am going to share with you the formula of food combinations that will help you reach your goal. Play with these, mixing and matching according to your taste. The important thing is that you keep your goal in mind. As you will see, you won't be eating boring, flavorless meals.

It is only 21 days. Take it day by day, and you will see how it becomes easier when the days go by and you start seeing results. I can assure you that after the first week, you will feel great and start to notice the difference in your clothes, your mood, your energy; it will be easier to stay focused on your goal. That is the whole idea: not giving up. It is a challenge that you can accomplish and enjoy the results *forever.*

Before jumping into food combinations, I want to give you three rules to guide your overall eating habits.

1. Never go more than three hours without eating. You must eat five to six times a day; three main meals and at least two snacks

in between. When you constantly eat, your body and your metabolism increase, aiding your digestion. When you stay on track and eat five to six small meals a day, you will burn the largest amount of calories. However, don't think that you can eat anything you want; it does not work like that!

2. Don't eat starchy carbohydrates after lunch—this is a fundamental rule. Some carbohydrates give you more energy than others, but they are also harder to burn. It is important to know the difference between good and bad carbohydrates. The good ones are really healthy for you because they provide the energy that your body needs. Without carbohydrates, you can't have good training sessions and your energy levels decrease, making you feel more tired during the day. The reality is that there is no good time to eat a bad carbohydrate. I will explain that in a minute!

3. Consider bad carbohydrates to equal white carbohydrates, flours, bread, white rice, etc. Even though good carbohydrates are excellent for you during the day and before training, you must avoid them after lunch. That way, they won't store in your body and turn into fat while you sleep at night. Having these two types of carbohydrates clear and knowing when to eat the good carbs helps a lot in the process of losing weight.

Don't let anyone tell you otherwise; you *must* eat carbohydrates. They will provide constant energy and they actually make you burn more fat at the gym. Just be careful with the types of carbohydrates that you eat!

ARE YOU READY?

Are you ready to start your 21 days to success?

This is the moment that you have been waiting for. From now on, we are going to use all the things that we have learned until now, and put them in action to *Kick-start the New You!*

This new you will be filled with energy and confidence. The new you is an image of perfect health, an image that also motivates everyone around you. You will be an inspiration to others who want to look as good and feel as wonderful as you do.

You are what you eat, and if you follow this formula, you will look amazing!

When you are in the process of planning your meals, I recommend you to follow these suggestions:

1. Whatever animal proteins that you choose to eat must be grilled, baked, barbecued, or steamed. To give them flavor, add some lemon, garlic, sea salt, and pepper.

2. The same goes for the vegetables; they must be seasoned with salt and pepper, preferably, sea salt. You can steam them with a little olive or grape oil.

3. Remember that the dressing for the salad should be homemade. An easy recipe: apple cider vinegar with olive oil, sea salt, and pepper.

4. It is important to drink water during the day; drink approximately 2 glasses with each meal.

5. Start your day with a cup warm water and half of a squeezed lemon to kick-start your metabolism and prepare the body to burn fat.

6. To get the most benefits and calm your cravings for more food, start your day with a tablespoon of chia seeds (soak them for 15 minutes in a glass of water before drinking it). You can use flaxseed, instead; also soak them for fifteen minutes and drink at least fifteen minutes before breakfast, and repeat at dinner.

7. If you are allergic to caffeine, consult your doctor or use decaffeinated green tea.

Note: These are recommendations. The information provided in this book is simply informative; it is not to be used as a substitute of your doctor's or nutritionist's advice. You must always consult with your doctor or health care provider about any doubts you may have about your health condition.

EAT BREAKFAST LIKE A KING

"Eat breakfast like a king," that's how the old saying goes. And even though a lot of people know this, they don't put it in action. They don't understand that this is the most important meal of the day.

The meaning is in its name, "breakfast": you *break* the *fast* that you've been in all night. Because, even if we are resting, our organs are working all those hours, using energy. So, getting back that energy is as easy as giving it a good dose of fuel through food.

A lot of people think that filling up with coffee or eating a banana or a doughnut is good enough; they call this a breakfast. But, in reality, their bodies will crash very soon, looking for more caffeine and food. When their bodies crash, the metabolism slows; they're not burning any fat, and so it's no wonder that they are not losing weight.

So, let's leave the bad habits and start our mornings with this new formula. Are you ready?

Breakfast Formula: Carbohydrates + Proteins + Fiber

For example: ½ cup oatmeal + egg omelet + ½ cup strawberries

MORNING SNACK

Now, let's go onto snacks.

As I've mentioned, to keep the metabolism moving, it is important to eat every three hours. This will help us keep our insulin levels up and keep the metabolism strong. So, here is the formula that you should follow for the morning snacks. Don't be afraid of including carbohydrates at this time; your body will use them as energy.

Morning Snack Formula: Carbohydrates + Fiber + Protein

For example: ¼ cup raw oatmeal + blue berries + 1 scoop of vanilla whey protein

EAT LUNCH LIKE A PRINCE

If you eat breakfast like a king, then you should eat lunch like a prince!

Note that we should not eliminate complex carbohydrates from our lunch, because these are a good source of energy that keeps feeding our bodies and helps them to stay full for longer. But be careful, you need to watch your portions. Eating carbs doesn't mean that you can eat a huge plate of food; instead, you should enjoy it in moderation. The appropriate amount is ½ cup for women and 1 cup for men. In formula terms, that means:

Lunch Formula: Carbohydrates + Protein + Fiber

For example: ½ cup brown rice + grilled chicken + green vegetables

"MAGIC HOUR": AFTERNOON SNACK

This is the most important time of the day. Many experts call it the "magic hour." It is around four in the afternoon, precisely in between lunch and dinner, and exactly when our insulin levels start to drop. One of the keys to staying fit and skinny is to avoid falling for snack machines. This is the time where you should eat some protein and fiber; this will help you stay full for longer. It also helps to move the metabolism and regulate insulin levels, helping us eat in moderation at dinner.

The secret formula is:

Afternoon Snack Formula: Protein + Fiber

For example: Plain Greek yogurt + raspberries + 1 Tbsp. honey

EAT DINNER LIKE A BEGGAR

This part of the old saying means that your dinner should be light. As we can see, after lunch, we avoid starchy carbohydrates and we focus on eating fiber and protein, since our bodies don't require that much energy to go to sleep. When we overeat, what we eat turns into sugar and from there into fat.

Dinner Formula: Protein + Fiber

For example: Grilled fish + broccoli

THE LAST SNACK

Some of us stay hungry, especially if we train or we have a very active day, so I recommend doing one last snack before going to bed. This will help you keep your metabolism moving and your muscles fed.

Evening Snack Formula: Protein

For example: protein shake, egg whites, Greek yogurt with flaxseed, or raw almonds

JUICES AND DRINKS

This is my present for you, to give you that extra push you need during these 21 days. Here are some of my favorite recipes for green juices and blends. You can use them as a snack, to help you to burn more fat, to accelerate your metabolism, to improve your digestion, and to strengthen your energy levels. These fat-burning green juices are a great way to complement your 21-day challenge and get the best results. Green juices will help detoxify your body by removing the fiber from the intestines and thus resting the digestive system. The body uses this energy to repair cells and remove toxins. Green juices have additional benefits including improving your complexion, improving your sleep quality, reducing pain, strengthening the immune system, and the best part— losing weight!

Juice to fight abdominal fat
Ingredients:

> 1 cup pineapple
>
> ½ cup aloe vera
>
> 1 tsp. of chia seeds or flaxseed
>
> 1 glass of water

Blend well and enjoy!

Alkaline, detoxifying, and slimming juice
Ingredients:

> 1 green apple
>
> 1 lemon, juiced
>
> ½ cucumber
>
> 1 celery stalk
>
> 1 chunk (2 cm.) of fresh ginger

Blend well and enjoy!

Juice to cleanse the colon

Ingredients:

> 1 Tbsp. chia seeds
>
> 2 apples
>
> 2 chard leaves

Blend well and enjoy! If it comes out too thick, add a little water. Drink it 3 times a day, for a week. Your intestines will feel the difference. Don't give up on this treatment. You will see bowel movements, soon enough, helping you to train your intestines, without medication.

Juice to control stomach bloating and end constipation

This juice is perfect for when you feel bloated. It helps with digestion and prevents other stomach problems.

Ingredients:

> 1 cup papaya
>
> 1 Tbsp. flaxseed
>
> 2 cups water
>
> 2 Tbsp. raw oatmeal
>
> 1 tsp. of honey

Blend well and enjoy! Drink it before breakfast for a week and enjoy all the benefits. It's amazing!

Juice to cleanse your liver and kidneys

Dill helps to cleanse the liver and kidneys in a natural way; it also improves digestion, reduces gas, and helps to lose weight.

Ingredients:

> 1 liter of water
>
> 1 bunch of dill
>
> 2 Tbsp. lemon juice
>
> 2 Tbsp. honey

Preparation: Let the dill soak for 15 minutes in water, then add the lemon juice and honey. Drink it daily.

Juice to fight cellulite

Ingredients:

> 2 celery stalks
>
> 1 bunch of parsley
>
> 1 carrot
>
> 1 apple
>
> 1 chunk (2 cm.) of ginger

Blend well and enjoy! Drink 2–3 times a week, in the morning.

Digestive and slimming juice

Ingredients:

> ½ grapefruit, juiced
>
> 1 pineapple slice
>
> 1 bunch of parsley
>
> 1 chunk (2 cm.) of ginger
>
> 1 chunk of aloe vera
>
> 1 Tbsp. flaxseed

Blend well and enjoy!

Chapter 12

21-DAY KICK-START MENU

You are on your way, and I'm sure that there will be no turning back for you. You have detoxified your body from all the junk that didn't let you lose weight, from all the toxins and food residues. You are now ready to start a real change! From now on, whatever goes in your mouth will have a purpose.

You will start to eat consciously, knowing that every food you eat is meant to energize you and burn fat. But what exactly should you eat? I want to give you a hand so that your next trip to the supermarket is different. You will go with a positive mind. Your top priority is losing weight and recovering your health. To make it easier for you, here is a list of products that you should have at home for the next 21 days. Take it with you and you will see that the process becomes much easier.

Cheer up! When you finally realize how fun and delicious your meals will be, you will be happy you made this decision. Even more, when you see the results on your body, your mood, your health, and your self-confidence, you will be ecstatic! So, let's do it!

Fruits:

- Apple (green or yellow)
- Avocado
- Blackberry
- Blueberry
- Cantaloupe
- Grapefruit
- Honeydew melon
- Kiwi
- Lemon and lime
- Mulberry
- Oranges
- Passion fruits
- Peach
- Plums
- Raspberry
- Strawberry

Vegetables:

- Artichoke
- Asparagus (white or green)
- Beet
- Bell pepper
- Broccoli
- Cabbage
- Carrot
- Cauliflower
- Celery
- Cilantro
- Eggplant
- Fennel
- Garlic
- Ginger
- Kale
- Lettuce
- Onion
- Parsley
- Pumpkin
- Radish
- Spinach
- Swiss chard
- Tomato
- Watercress

Carbohydrates:

- Sweet potato

Proteins:

- Almond butter
- Beans
- Chickpeas
- Chicken breast
- Egg whites
- Lentils
- Low-sugar jam
- Peanut butter
- Salmon
- Tuna in water
- Turkey breast
- Whey protein
- White fish (cod or pollock)

Whole wheat products:

- Brown pasta
- Brown rice
- Oatmeal
- Quinoa
- Rice puff cakes
- Wheat germ
- Whole wheat bread or Ezekiel bread
- Whole wheat crackers
- Whole wheat tortillas

Dressings:

- Apple cider vinegar
- Balsamic vinegar
- Greek yogurt or plain yogurt
- Honey
- Olive oil
- Rice vinegar
- Sesame oil

Other:

- Almond milk
- Cinnamon
- Coconut milk
- Coconut water
- Green tea, red or herbal tea, decaffeinated
- Oolong tea
- Pepper
- Sea salt

Seeds and super foods:

- Almonds (or raw walnuts, no salt)
- Brazil nuts
- Chia seeds
- Flaxseed
- Goji berries
- Hemp seeds
- Peanuts (no salt)
- Pumpkin seeds
- Red berries or raisins
- Sunflower seeds

RECIPES

It's so great to be part of your transformation journey! I know that sometimes we don't have enough time or we simply have too much to do to think about what's for supper. Sometimes, the mind goes blank when it comes to thinking up easy, quick, delicious, and healthy meals. So I just wanted to surprise you. I want to give you 21 recipes for breakfast, lunch, dinner, and snacks, to make this a lot easier for you.

With these recipes, you can complete 21 days, the magic, wholesome number to get to the new habit of eating healthy and to kick-start the *new you* who is filled with energy. You can mix and match as you like with these recipes. That way you won't get bored, and you will always be able to find a way to eat in a healthy, easy, and delicious way. Be creative, but also stay true to your goals and yourself. Just remember to follow the appropriate portions and food formula discussed in the previous chapter.

BREAKFASTS

1. Veggie Omelet

Ingredients:

> 3 egg whites
>
> 1 whole egg
>
> ½ tomato
>
> 1 bunch of spinach
>
> 2 slices of Ezekiel or P28 bread (or any whole wheat bread)
>
> ⅓ pineapple, cubed

Preparation: Spray non-stick cooking oil on a pan and pour the egg mixture with the vegetables. Cook until it is set on the edges and halfway in the middle when nudged with a spatula. Serve with bread and cubed pineapple.

2. Oatmeal Breakfast Cake with Apples and Strawberries

Ingredients:

> ½ cup raw oatmeal
>
> 4 egg whites
>
> ¼ cup pumpkin puree
>
> ¼ cup shredded coconut
>
> ½ scoop of vanilla whey protein
>
> ¼ tsp. of baking powder
>
> ¼ tsp. of cinnamon powder
>
> ½ green apple
>
> 5 strawberries, sliced

Preparation: In a microwave-safe bowl, mix the oatmeal, egg whites, pumpkin puree, shredded coconut, protein powder, and baking powder. Microwave for 5–6 minutes or until cooked. With the help of a knife or a spatula, separate the cake from the pan, turn over onto a plate, add the apple and strawberry slices, and drizzle some honey on top to serve.

3. Healthy "Huevos Rancheros"

Ingredients:

>2 whole eggs
>
>2 egg whites
>
>2 Tbsp. fresh salsa (see below)
>
>½ avocado
>
>1 slice Ezekiel (or whole wheat) bread

Preparation: Spray the bottom of heated pan with oil to "fry" the eggs. Serve the eggs with 2 Tbsp. fresh salsa, a toasted slice of bread and ½ of a small avocado.

Fresh Salsa

Ingredients:

>2 tomatoes
>
>1 onion
>
>2 limes
>
>1 garlic clove
>
>1 bunch of cilantro
>
>Sea salt and pepper to taste
>
>1 small jalapeño pepper (optional)

Preparation: Chop the tomatoes, onion, garlic, cilantro leaves, and jalapeño. Juice the limes and add sea salt and pepper to taste and mix well.

You can store the salsa in a glass container in the fridge for up to a week!

4. Pumpkin and Protein Pancakes

Ingredients:

> ½ cup pumpkin puree
>
> 3 egg whites
>
> ¼ cup oatmeal flour
>
> ⅓ tsp. baking powder
>
> 1 Tbsp. pumpkin pie spice
>
> 4 fresh strawberries, sliced
>
> 1 Tbsp. maple syrup

Preparation: Mix the puree, flour, egg whites, pumpkin spice, and baking powder. In a previously heated pan, add the mixture and cook the pancake for about 3 minutes on each side, until golden. Serve on a plate; add the strawberries and the syrup. Enjoy!

5. Veggie Omelet

Ingredients:

> 1 whole egg
>
> 3 egg whites
>
> ¼ cup cooked broccoli
>
> ¼ cup mushrooms, chopped
>
> ¼ onion, chopped
>
> 1 tomato, chopped
>
> Sea salt and pepper to taste

Preparation: In a bowl, mix the eggs and chopped veggies and season with sea salt and pepper to taste. In a heated pan, spray some oil and add the egg mixture. When the eggs start to bubble, fold them in half with the help of a spatula, cover the pan, and let it cook for 3–4 minutes. I serve them with half a grapefruit.

6. Energy Booster Breakfast

Ingredients:

> ½ cup frozen acai berries
>
> ⅓ cup strawberries, sliced
>
> ⅓ cup raspberries
>
> ⅓ cup blueberries
>
> ⅓ cup oatmeal, cooked
>
> 2 Tbsp. desiccated coconut
>
> 2 Tbsp. goji berries
>
> 2 Tbsp. honey

Preparation: In a small bowl, pour the cooked oatmeal. Add all the fruits on top and drizzle with honey.

7. Very Berry Oatmeal

Ingredients:

> ⅓ cup oatmeal
>
> 2 egg whites
>
> ⅔ cup water
>
> 1 Tbsp. honey
>
> 1 cup mixed berries
>
> ¼ cup sliced almonds
>
> Dash of cinnamon

Preparation: In a small pot over medium heat, add the oatmeal and water; stir. When its consistency starts to change, add the egg whites and mix until incorporated, turn off the heat and add the almonds, cinnamon, and honey. Serve with fresh berries.

8. Blueberry Pancakes

Ingredients:

> ¾ cup almond flour
>
> ½ cup oatmeal flour
>
> ¼ tsp. baking soda
>
> 1 tsp. baking powder
>
> 1 cup Greek yogurt
>
> 2 Tbsp. apple compote or marmalade with no sugar
>
> 2 Tbsp. almond milk
>
> 1 egg
>
> 1 cup fresh blueberries

Preparation: Add almond flour, oatmeal, baking soda, baking powder, Greek yogurt, almond milk, apple compote or marmalade, and egg to a blender and blend until smooth. Spray with cooking spray the bottom of a hot pan, pour the mixture to cook the pancakes until golden brown on each side. Serve with fresh blueberries and a drizzle of honey.

9. Breakfast Barley

Ingredients:

> ½ cup cooked barley
>
> 1 Tbsp. homemade peanut butter
>
> 1 Tbsp. chia seeds
>
> ⅓ cup coconut or almond milk
>
> 1 Tbsp. pumpkin pie spice or cinnamon
>
> 1 handful of walnuts
>
> 1 handful of cranberries or raisins
>
> 1 tsp. of honey

Preparation: In a pot over medium heat, add the barley, coconut, or almond milk, chia seeds and pumpkin spice or cinnamon; mix well until its consistency changes. Serve with the cranberries or raisins, walnuts, and honey; top with peanut butter.

For the Barley

In a pot over high heat, add 1 cup barley and 3 cups water; let it boil, cover and lower the heat. Let it cook for 45 minutes to an hour over low heat. Tip: Soaking the barley the night before will reduce the cooking time, and it'll be easier to digest.

10. Chocolate Oatmeal with Strawberries and Kiwi

Ingredients:

> ½ cup oatmeal
>
> 1 cup water
>
> 1 scoop of whey protein chocolate flavor
>
> 5 strawberries, sliced
>
> 1 kiwi, cubed

Preparation: In a pot over medium heat, add the oatmeal and the water; mix until it thickens, lower the heat, and add the chocolate protein powder. Serve with the sliced strawberries and kiwi.

11. Tropical Breakfast

Ingredients:

> ½ cup coconut milk
>
> 1 Tbsp. honey
>
> 4 drops vanilla extract
>
> ⅓ cup chia seed
>
> ¼ cup nuts or almonds
>
> 1 Tbsp. desiccated coconut
>
> ½ cup berries or other fresh fruits of your choice

Preparation: In a small mixing bowl combine the coconut milk, honey, and chia seeds. Use plastic wrapping paper to cover the bowl and refrigerate during night or at least 45 minutes before adding the rest of the ingredients. Serve in a small, deep plate and add the berries on top; refrigerate for another 20 minutes and enjoy!

12. Asparagus Egg Omelet

Ingredients:

> 1 egg
>
> 3 egg whites
>
> 5 asparagus
>
> 1 bunch of spinach leaves
>
> ¼ small onion, chopped
>
> 2 Tbsp. fresh salsa (see page 154)

Preparation: Mix the egg and the egg whites. Spray the bottom of a heated pan with cooking spray, sauté the onions; chop the asparagus and add them to the pan, cook for a minute, add the spinach leaves and stir. Add the eggs and cover the pan, lower the heat and cook for about 4 minutes or until set. Serve the egg omelet with two tablespoons of fresh salsa.

13. Veggie Egg Burrito

Ingredients:

> 1 egg
>
> 2 egg whites
>
> A handful of spinach leaves
>
> ⅓ cup mushrooms, sliced
>
> ¼ small onion, chopped
>
> 1 whole grain 8-inch tortilla
>
> ¼ of an avocado
>
> Sea salt and pepper

Preparation: In a bowl mix the eggs. Spray a heated pan with cooking oil. Add the onions and cook for a couple of minutes; when they become translucent, add the sliced mushroom. Add the eggs and scramble, when the eggs are almost ready, add the spinach leaves and finish cooking. Serve on the warm whole grain tortilla, top with avocado slices, and fold like a burrito.

14. Piña Colada Oatmeal

Ingredients:

> ½ cup oatmeal
>
> 1 cup water
>
> ½ cup coconut milk
>
> 2 egg whites
>
> 2 Tbsp. shredded coconut
>
> 1 Tbsp. honey
>
> ¼ cup chopped pineapple
>
> 1 strawberry
>
> A pinch of cinnamon

Preparation: To a pot over medium heat add the oatmeal, coconut milk, and water; mix well and add the egg whites; continue mixing until it thickens, about 3 minutes. Turn off the heat and add the cinnamon and shredded coconut, mix, and serve topped with the fresh strawberry and pineapple.

15. Waffle and Peanut Butter Breakfast

Ingredients

> 1 whole wheat waffle (see below)
> 1 Tbsp. peanut butter
> 1 Tbsp. honey
> ⅓ cup blueberries
> ½ grapefruit
> 2 Tbsp. raw flaked almonds

Whole Wheat Waffle Ingredients: (Serves 4)

> 1 egg
> 1 cup whole wheat flour
> 2 Tbsp. coconut oil
> 1 Tbsp. Stevia (optional)
> 1 Tbsp. baking powder
> ½ Tbsp. vanilla

Preparation: Mix all the whole wheat waffle ingredients in a small mixing bowl until combined. Pour the mixture in a waffle iron and cook for 5 minutes; transfer to a plate. Spread 1 tablespoon of peanut butter on the waffle and put the blueberries on top. Drizzle honey and sprinkle almonds on top. Serve with half a grapefruit.

16. Turkey Omelet

Ingredients:

> 1 egg
>
> 3 egg whites
>
> ¼ cup ground turkey meat
>
> 1 tomato, chopped
>
> ¼ small onion, chopped
>
> 1 garlic clove, chopped
>
> Sea salt and pepper
>
> ½ grapefruit

Preparation: In a heated pan, add a bit of coconut oil to coat, add the chopped onions and cook for a minute; add the ground turkey, garlic, and sea salt and pepper, continue to cook and add the tomatoes. In a bowl, mix the egg and the egg whites, add the eggs to the pan, lower the heat and cover to cook for about 5 more minutes until the eggs look done. Serve with half a grapefruit.

17. Oatmeal and Cottage Cheese Pancakes

Ingredients:

> ½ cup oatmeal
>
> ⅓ cup cottage cheese
>
> 2 eggs
>
> Dash of cinnamon
>
> 1 tsp. vanilla extract
>
> 1 Tbsp. honey
>
> ½ cup strawberries, sliced

Preparation: In a blender add the oatmeal, cottage cheese, eggs, cinnamon, and vanilla extract and blend. In a heated pan coated with a little coconut oil, pour the mixture to cook the pancakes, cook until golden brown on both sides. Serve with the fresh strawberries and drizzle with honey.

18. Greek Yogurt with Fruit Salad

Ingredients:

> 1 cup mixed fruits: mango, grapes, strawberries, grapefruit
>
> ⅓ cup Greek yogurt or natural plain yogurt
>
> 1 handful of walnuts (no salt)
>
> 1 Tbsp. honey

Preparation: Chop the fruit into bite size pieces, chop the walnuts, mix with the Greek natural yogurt, and drizzle honey on top.

19. Oatmeal with In-Season Fruits

Ingredients:

> ½ cup oatmeal
>
> ⅓ cup egg whites
>
> 1 cup water
>
> 1 pinch of cinnamon
>
> 1 Tbsp. honey
>
> 1 peach
>
> 5 strawberries, sliced

Preparation: Cook the oatmeal with the egg whites, water, and cinnamon, for about 3 minutes, stirring. Once it is ready, add the honey, cut the fruit, and enjoy.

20. French Toast with Fresh Strawberries

Ingredients:

> 2 slices of Ezekiel (or whole wheat) bread
>
> 4 egg whites
>
> A pinch of cinnamon
>
> 6 strawberries, sliced
>
> 1 Tbsp. honey

Preparation: Spray the bottom of a heated pan with coconut oil; mix the eggs and cinnamon, and soak the bread in it; let some of the excess drip off and place the bread on the heated pan, cook until golden brown on both sides. Serve with some powdered cinnamon, fresh strawberries, and a drizzle of honey.

21. Brown Rice and Egg Omelet

Ingredients:

> 1 whole egg
>
> 3 egg whites
>
> ¼ red onion, chopped
>
> 1 celery stalk, chopped
>
> 4 Tbsp. cooked brown rice (see below)
>
> 2 Tbsp. fresh salsa (see page 154)
>
> 1 slice of Ezekiel (or whole grain) bread
>
> ¼ cup blueberries

Preparation: In a bowl mix the eggs, brown rice, and vegetables. Add the mixture to a heated pan and let it cook for about 2 minutes, fold the eggs in half with a spatula, cover, and continue to cook for about 4 minutes. Serve with a slice of Ezekiel or whole grain bread and fresh blueberries.

Brown Rice

> 1 cup brown rice
>
> 2 ¼ cups water
>
> 1 onion, chopped
>
> 1 Tbsp. grape oil or olive oil
>
> Sea salt and pepper to taste

Preparation: In a pan, add the oil and sauté the onion, and then add the water and the previously washed and drained rice. Add sea salt and pepper and let it come to a boil, and then reduce the heat to a minimum for 45 minutes (covered). Take a look, and if it still looks hard, add a little more water, and follow this process until it looks soft and spongy. Some people put it in a pressure pot which softens it and then let it rest for a while before cooking it.

SNACKS

1. Peanut Butter and Ezekiel Bread

Ingredients:

> 1 slice of Ezekiel (or whole wheat) bread
>
> 1 Tbsp. peanut butter
>
> 1 Tbsp. honey

Preparation: Spread the peanut butter on the bread and drizzle with the honey.

2. Peanuts and Fresh Fruit

Ingredients:

> ¼ cup peanuts (no salt added)
>
> 1 cubed pear

Preparation: Add the ingredients together in a bowl and enjoy.

3. Greek Yogurt and Strawberries

Ingredients:

> ½ cup Greek yogurt
> ⅓ cup strawberries
> 1 Tbsp. honey

Preparation: Mix the yogurt with the strawberries and add the honey.

4. Eggs and Green Apple

Ingredients:

> 1 hardboiled egg
> 1 green apple

Preparation: It's as simple as it sounds; place the ingredients onto a plate and enjoy!

5. Chocolate Protein Pudding

Ingredients:

> 1 Tbsp. chocolate protein pudding
> ½ cup Greek yogurt

Preparation: Mix well and enjoy!

6. Avocado and Egg Sandwich

Ingredients:

> 1 slice of Ezekiel or whole wheat bread
> ¼ avocado, pureed
> 1 hardboiled egg, sliced
> Sea salt and pepper

Preparation: Spread the puree on the bread. Add the egg on top, season with sea salt and pepper.

7. Cottage Cheese and Salmon

Ingredients:

> 2 rice cakes
>
> 2 Tbsp. ricotta
>
> 2 slices of smoked salmon

Preparation: Spread the cottage cheese on the rice cakes, and top with smoked salmon. Season with sea salt and pepper.

8. Refreshing Juice

Ingredients:

> ½ cucumber
>
> 2 celery stalks
>
> 1 pineapple slice
>
> 1 bunch of parsley
>
> 1 Tbsp. chia seeds
>
> 2 cups cold water

Preparation: Blend and enjoy with the almonds on the side.

9. Peanut Butter and Chocolate Balls

Ingredients:

> ¼ cup peanut butter
>
> ¼ cup raw oatmeal
>
> 1 scoop of chocolate whey protein
>
> 1 tsp. of honey

Preparation: In a bowl, mix the peanut butter, whey protein, and honey; form into balls, place in the fridge for 20 minutes, and enjoy. (Extras can be refrigerated for later!)

10. Antioxidant Protein Shake

Ingredients:

> 1 cup almond milk
>
> ½ cup raspberries or blueberries
>
> 1 scoop of whey protein

Preparation: Blend well and enjoy!

11. Apple and Almond

Ingredients:

> 1 green apple, sliced
>
> 2 Tbsp. almond butter
>
> 1 Tbsp. honey

Preparation: Place the apple in a bowl, add the almond butter, and drizzle with honey.

12. Edamame Beans

Ingredients:

> 1 cup edamame with sea salt
>
> 1 cup green tea

Preparation: Microwave the edamame for a minute and enjoy with your green tea.

13. Veggies and Dip

Ingredients:

> 2 carrots, sliced
>
> 1 celery stalk, sliced
>
> ¼ cup plain Greek yogurt
>
> 1 garlic clove, minced
>
> 1 tsp. lemon juice

Preparation: Mix the garlic with the lemon juice and the yogurt, enjoy with some veggie sticks!

14. Mega-Berry Shake

Ingredients:

> 1 scoop of whey protein
>
> ¼ cup blueberries
>
> ¼ cup raspberries
>
> 1 Tbsp. chia seeds
>
> 1 cup coconut water
>
> 1 pinch of cinnamon
>
> 1 cup water

Preparation: Blend for a minute and enjoy!

15. Rice Cake with Toppings

Ingredients:

> 1 rice cake
>
> 1 Tbsp. peanut butter
>
> ¼ cup of shredded coconut
>
> ¼ cup berries of your choice

Preparation: Spread the peanut butter onto the rice cake; add the berries, then the coconut.

16. Ants on a Log

Ingredients:

> 2 celery stalks
>
> 1 Tbsp. peanut butter
>
> 1 small bunch of raisins

Preparation: Cut the celery into thumb-size pieces. Fill with the peanut butter, add the raisins.

17. Tropical Shake

Ingredients:

> 2 pineapple slices
>
> 1 lemon, juiced
>
> 1 chunk of ginger (2 cm.)
>
> 1 scoop of whey protein
>
> 1 pinch of cinnamon
>
> 2 cups water

Preparation: Blend well and enjoy!

18. Cottage Cheese with Strawberries

Ingredients:

> ⅓ cup cottage cheese
>
> 1 Tbsp. chia seeds
>
> ⅓ cup strawberries
>
> 1 Tbsp. honey

Preparation: Mix the cottage cheese with the chia seeds. Then, add the strawberries and drizzle with honey.

19. Whole Wheat Rice Cracker with Almond Butter and Strawberries

Ingredients:

      1 whole wheat rice cake

      2 Tbsp. almond or peanut butter

      1 Tbsp. honey

      3 chopped strawberries

Preparation: Spread the butter on the rice cake, add the strawberries, and drizzle with honey.

*Note: You can buy these rice cakes in any supermarket. They are very low in calories and excellent for snacks. If you don't find them, you can use a slice of whole wheat bread instead.

20. Brazil Nuts with Cranberries

Ingredients:

      ¼ cup Brazil nuts

      ¼ cup cranberries

*Note: Brazil nuts contain essential polyunsaturated fatty acids, primarily linoleic. They contain vitamin E and also A and C, some of the B complex, and also selenium, which makes them antioxidants. They are great for fighting cravings because they're high in protein and good fats.

21. Mango, Strawberry, and Walnut Salad

Ingredients:

      ½ cup mango and strawberry

      ⅓ cup plain, no sugar added, Greek yogurt

      ¼ cup walnuts

Preparation: Mix well and enjoy!

LUNCHES

1. Tuna Salad

Ingredients:

>   1 cup brown rice, cooked (see page 165)
>   ½ cup tuna
>   ½ onion, chopped
>   A splash of olive oil
>   1 bunch of cilantro
>   Sea salt and pepper to taste
>   1 cup leafy greens

Preparation: Chop the onion and cilantro; drain the water from the canned tuna, and mix the ingredients. Place the tuna on top of a bed of leafy greens and put the rice on the side.

2. Vegan Lunch: Lentils and Rice

Ingredients:

>   2 Tbsp. olive oil
>   3 medium sized carrots, chopped
>   1 medium sized onion, chopped
>   1 tsp. of fresh garlic
>   ¼ tsp. of sea salt
>   ¼ tsp. of freshly ground black pepper
>   1 cup organic lentils, washed and drained
>   2 chopped tomatoes
>   ½ cup cooked brown rice (see page 165)

Preparation: In a pan, sauté onion, and garlic until cooked, then add the carrots and tomatoes and cook a few more minutes. Once the vegetables are cooked, add the previously washed and drained lentils, add sea salt and pepper and the water. Bring to a boil and lower the temperature to low; cook for 20 minutes or until the lentils are soft.

3. Portobello Burger

Ingredients:

> 2 Portobello mushrooms
>
> 5 oz. chicken breast
>
> 2 Tbsp. guacamole (see below)
>
> Paprika
>
> 1 garlic clove
>
> Sea salt and pepper
>
> 1 cup fresh vegetables of your choice

Preparation: Season the chicken breast with the garlic, paprika, sea salt and pepper. Grill for 20 minutes. Grab the Portobello mushrooms and grill them for 5 minutes. When they're done, build your burger using the mushrooms as bread buns and guacamole as a substitute for ketchup and mayonnaise. Serve with a fresh vegetable as a side.

Guacamole

Ingredients:

> 1 small avocado
>
> ¼ small red onion, chopped
>
> 1 tomato, chopped
>
> 1 lemon or lime, juiced
>
> Sea salt and pepper to taste

Preparation: In a bowl, puree avocado with a fork; add the lemon, onions and tomato, season with sea salt and pepper and mix well.

4. Chicken Wrap

Ingredients:

>4 oz. chicken breast, julienned
>
>½ yellow pepper, julienned
>
>½ red pepper, julienned
>
>½ white onion, julienned
>
>⅓ cup pico de gallo (see below)
>
>1 whole wheat tortilla
>
>½ small avocado

Preparation: In a pan, add a splash of olive oil and heat until smoking, then add the chicken with the julienned onion and pepper. Stir continuously for 5 minutes. Season with sea salt and pepper. Roll up the chicken and vegetable mixture in your wrap; cut diagonally in half. Serve with pico de gallo and avocado.

Pico de Gallo:

>½ peeled tomatoes chopped in small cubes
>
>1 Tbsp. white onion, diced
>
>1 Tbsp. green onion, chopped
>
>1 Tbsp. coriander, minced
>
>½ lime, juiced
>
>Sea salt and pepper

5. Chicken Fajitas

Ingredients:

> 2 whole wheat tortillas (6-inch)
>
> 6 oz. of chicken
>
> ½ red bell pepper
>
> ½ yellow bell pepper
>
> ½ white onion
>
> A little bit of grape oil
>
> Sea salt and pepper to taste
>
> ¼ cup black beans (previously cooked)
>
> ½ cup guacamole (see page 173)

Preparation: In a pan, sauté the peppers, onion, chicken, and sea salt and pepper to taste. Let it cook at a low heat. When done, put in fajita with fresh guacamole and enjoy!

6. Chicken Soup

Ingredients:

> 1 skinless, boneless chicken breast
>
> 1 chunk of pumpkin
>
> 1 onion
>
> 3 celery stalks
>
> 2 carrots
>
> ¼ cup low-sodium tomato paste
>
> Sea salt and pepper to taste
>
> ½ cup previously cooked brown rice (see page 165)

Preparation: In a pan with water, cook the chicken for about 20 minutes, add sea salt. Then, add the rest of the ingredients for about 30 minutes more. Shred the chicken, add the cilantro, and enjoy with rice!

7. Tuna Wrap

Ingredients:

> 1 whole wheat tortilla (8-inch)
>
> 1 Tbsp. hummus
>
> ½ cup tuna in water, drained
>
> ½ red onion
>
> 1 celery stalk
>
> 1 Tbsp. grape oil
>
> Sea salt and pepper to taste
>
> Romaine lettuce
>
> ¼ cup cabbage
>
> 2 Tbsp. sesame oil
>
> 2 Tbsp. rice vinegar
>
> 1 Tbsp. soy sauce

Preparation: Chop the onion and celery, add the grape oil, and mix in the tuna. On the tortilla, add the hummus; then the lettuce, then the tuna on top and roll it up. On the side, cut the cabbage thinly, add oil, vinegar, and soy sauce.

8. Chicken Done Simple

Ingredients:

> 5 oz. of chicken breast
>
> 1 tomato
>
> ½ onion
>
> ½ sweet potato
>
> 1 bunch of spinach
>
> Olive oil
>
> Sea salt and pepper, to taste

Preparation: Cut the sweet potato in squares, add 1 tsp. olive oil, and bake in a preheated oven at 350° for 15 minutes or until soft.

Grill the chicken, season to taste with sea salt and pepper, and cut into squares when done. Salad: Mix the tomato, onion, and spinach. Add olive oil and season with sea salt and pepper.

9. Asparagus Soup with Quinoa Salad

Ingredients for Asparagus Soup:

> 10 asparagus stalks
>
> 2 cups water
>
> ½ onion, chopped
>
> ½ carrot, chopped
>
> ½ celery stalk, chopped
>
> Sea salt and pepper to taste

Preparation: Place all the ingredients in a saucepan until it boils, remove from the heat when tender, and let cool. Then, carefully blend for 60 seconds and enjoy!

Ingredients for Quinoa Salad:

> 1 cup quinoa
>
> 1 ½ cups water
>
> 1 bunch parsley
>
> 1 carrot, sliced thin
>
> 1 celery stalk, sliced thin
>
> 2 Tbsp. olive oil
>
> Sea salt to taste
>
> 3 limes

Preparation: Wash the quinoa three times before cooking. Place it in a pan with water, and bring to a boil; then lower the heat until the water evaporates. Squeeze a lime to give it more consistency (it takes about 20–25 minutes to cook). Remove from the heat; keep the pan covered until cool. Add the rest of the chopped vegetables, the juice of 2 limes, olive oil, and sea salt to taste.

10. Tuna Sandwich with Salad

Ingredients:

    2 slices of Ezekiel (or whole wheat) bread

    1 can of tuna, in water, drained

    ½ onion, chopped

    1 Tbsp. olive oil

    1 lime

    Sea salt and pepper to taste

    2 cups arugula

    Vinaigrette (sea salt, lime juice, olive oil, vinegar)

    ½ grapefruit

Preparation: Mix tuna with onion, olive oil, juice of 1 lime, and season with sea salt and pepper. Tuck in between two slices of bread. Mix the ingredients for the vinaigrette and add it on top of the arugula and grapefruit.

11. Baked Chicken with Sweet Potato

Ingredients:

    5 oz. chicken breast

    1 sweet potato

    1 zucchini, sliced

    Sea salt and pepper to taste

    Paprika

Preparation: Marinate the chicken breast with paprika, sea salt, and pepper. Cut the sweet potatoes into strips and place them with the zucchini and the chicken in an oven-safe dish. Bake for 25–30 minutes in the oven.

12. Ceviche with Sweet Potato

Ingredients:

> 6 oz. corvine or another fresh white fish
>
> 3 limes, juiced
>
> ½ of red onion, chopped
>
> 1 medium tomato, chopped
>
> Sea salt and pepper to taste
>
> ½ big sweet potato or 1 small
>
> Romaine lettuce

Salad Dressing:

> ½ tsp. honey, 1 tsp. mustard, 1 tsp. lime juice

Preparation: Cut the fish into cubes, add the lime juice, sea salt, chopped onion, and tomato; mix, cover and refrigerate for 20 minutes. Preheat the oven; cut the potato, season with sea salt, pepper, and a little olive oil, put on baking sheet. Bake at 350° for 15 minutes or until soft. Cut the lettuce or another leafy green and add a dressing made with honey, mustard, and lime.

13. Spaghetti Bolognese

Ingredients:

> 1 cup whole wheat spaghetti
>
> 6 oz. of ground turkey
>
> 1 medium tomato
>
> ½ onion
>
> 1 garlic clove
>
> Sea salt and pepper to taste

Preparation: Sauté onion, garlic and tomato, add the turkey, season to taste and cook until done. Cook the spaghetti following the instructions from the package, then mix in with the sauce.

14. Fish with Rice

Ingredients:

> 4 oz. cod or Alaskan pollock
>
> ½ yellow zucchini, julienned
>
> ½ green zucchini, julienned
>
> 1 scoop pico de gallo (see page 174)

Preparation: Season fish with lime juice and pepper. Preheat oven to 350° and bake the fish for 20 minutes. In a hot pan, spray cooking oil and sauté the zucchini for 5 minutes until golden. Remove from heat and thread onto a wooden skewer or place directly on plate.

15. Fish with Sweet Potato and Salad

Ingredients:

> 6 oz. of your favorite white fish
>
> ½ of a big sweet potato or 1 small
>
> 1–2 cups spinach
>
> 2 Tbsp. fresh salsa (see page 154)

Preparation: Preheat the oven to 350°; cut the sweet potato, season with sea salt, pepper, and a little olive oil. Bake for 15 minutes or until soft. In a previously heated pan, add a little coconut or grape oil and cook the fish. Dress the spinach with balsamic vinegar and place onto the plate with cooked fish and baked potato.

16. Salmon, Brown Rice, and Salad

Ingredients:

> 6 oz. of fresh salmon
>
> 2 cups spinach
>
> ½ cup mixed berries
>
> ½ cup brown rice, cooked (see page 165)

Preparation: In a preheated pan, cook the salmon in olive oil. While the salmon cooks, cut the fresh berries, and mix in with the spinach. Dress with olive oil, sea salt, pepper, and lime juice.

17. Chicken, French Fries, and Broccoli

Ingredients:

> 6 oz. of chicken breast, sliced
>
> 1 cup broccoli
>
> ½ sweet potato
>
> Sea salt and pepper to taste

Preparation: Preheat the oven; slice the sweet potato, season with sea salt and pepper, and a little olive oil. Bake at 350° for 15 minutes or until soft. While it is baking, season the chicken with sea salt and pepper and sauté in olive oil. On the side, steam the broccoli for 10 minutes or until soft.

18. Pasta with Ground Turkey

Ingredients:

> ½ cup uncooked whole wheat pasta
>
> 6 oz. of ground turkey
>
> 1 tomato
>
> 1 onion
>
> 1 pepper
>
> 1 cup broccoli
>
> 1 pinch of cayenne pepper
>
> Sea salt and black pepper to taste

Preparation: In a pan, sauté red onion, broccoli, and chopped tomato; add the turkey and cook at medium heat for 10 minutes. On the side, cook the pasta. Once all is ready, mix the sauce with the pasta.

19. Shredded Chicken Breast with Brown Rice and Avocado Salad

Ingredients:

> 5 oz. of chicken breast
>
> 1 medium tomato, diced
>
> 1 onion, diced
>
> 1 clove garlic, minced
>
> ½ cup cooked brown rice (see page 165)
>
> 2 cups green lettuce
>
> ½ avocado

Dressing:

> 1 Tbsp. grape oil or olive oil
>
> 2 Tbsp. vinegar
>
> Sea salt and pepper

Preparation: Boil the chicken breast in water with a little sea salt; remove and shred. Then cook with tomato, onion, garlic in a little grape oil. Once it is ready, serve it with ½ cup rice and avocado. You can add onions and tomatoes to the salad.

20. Quinoa Salad

Ingredients:

> 1 cup quinoa
>
> 1 ½ cups water
>
> 1 bunch of parsley
>
> 1 carrot
>
> 2 Tbsp. grape oil or olive oil
>
> Sea salt to taste
>
> 3 lemons
>
> ½ cup chopped almonds
>
> 2 cups arugula

Preparation: Wash the quinoa 3 times before cooking; place it in a pan with the water, and bring to a boil, then lower heat until the water evaporates. Squeeze a lemon to give it more consistency. Cook for 20–25 minutes. Then remove from heat; keep the pan covered until it cools down. Add the rest of the veggies, the juice of the two extra lemons, grape oil, sea salt, and parsley. Enjoy!

*Note: You can add some chickpeas or beans, if you don't like almonds.

21. Guilt-free Lunch

Ingredients

1 cod or Alaskan pollock fillet

4 oz. Japanese sweet potato, julienned and baked

6 endive leaves

1 garlic clove

1 Tbsp. coriander, minced

½ lemon, juiced

½ small avocado

Sea salt and pepper

Preparation: Season fish with sea salt, pepper, and garlic. Heat a non-stick pan, spray some cooking oil and add the fish. Cook for 8 minutes until golden on both sides. Remove from heat, cut into pieces, and fill up the endives. Place the avocado in a small bowl and add the lemon juice. Use a fork to mash, and then place on top of the filled endive leaves. Serve with baked Japanese sweet potato.

DINNERS

1. Tuna Salad

Ingredients:

> ½ cup canned tuna in water, drained
> ½ cup shredded carrot
> ½ cup shredded cucumber
> 1–2 cups spinach

Tuna:

> ½ onion, chopped
> 1–2 celery stalks
> 1 Tbsp. olive oil
> Sea salt and pepper to taste

Dressing:

> 1 Tbsp. sesame oil
> 1 Tbsp. rice vinegar
> 1 Tbsp. amino sauce or low-sodium soy sauce

Preparation: Chop the onions and celery, mix in with the tuna, and add olive oil, sea salt, and pepper to taste. Make a bed of spinach, add the shredded carrot and cucumber; then, add the tuna on top.

2. Grilled Chicken and Green Salad

Ingredients:

> 1–2 cups leafy greens
>
> 1 cucumber
>
> 6 oz. of chicken
>
> Sea salt and pepper
>
> 1 Tbsp. olive oil
>
> 1 Tbsp. apple cider vinegar
>
> 1 lemon or lime, juiced

Preparation: In a heated pan, cook the chicken with a little grape or coconut oil, sea salt, and pepper. While the chicken cooks, cut the cucumber and place it on top of a bed of leafy greens. Dressing: Mix the olive oil, vinegar, lemon or lime juice, sea salt, and pepper to taste.

3. Cream of Asparagus Soup

Ingredients:

> 1 bunch of asparagus
>
> 1 medium onion, chopped
>
> 2 or 3 garlic cloves
>
> Water
>
> Sea salt and pepper

Preparation: In a heated pot, sauté the onion with a little olive oil; after a few minutes add the chopped asparagus and the garlic, season with sea salt and pepper; add the water and cook over high heat until it starts to boil. Lower the heat and cook for 10 more minutes. Blend together.

4. Tuna Burgers with Green Salad, Avocado, and Fresh Salsa

Ingredients:

> 1 can of tuna in water, drained
>
> 1 onion
>
> 1 celery stalk
>
> 1 egg
>
> Sea salt and pepper
>
> 1–2 cups mixed lettuce
>
> ½ avocado
>
> ½ medium tomato
>
> 1 bunch of cilantro
>
> 1 lime, juiced

Preparation: Chop ½ onion and the celery. Mix in the egg, sea salt, pepper and the tuna. Form into patties, and cook briefly on medium heat; 30–60 seconds on each side. Cut the avocado, place it on top of a bed of lettuce, and dress with olive oil, sea salt, pepper, and apple cider vinegar. Fresh salsa: Chop ½ onion, tomato, cilantro; mix together, dress with olive oil, sea salt, pepper, and the juice of a lime.

5. Chicken and Salad

Ingredients:

> 6 oz. of chicken breast
>
> 1 bunch of parsley
>
> 1 garlic clove
>
> ½ avocado
>
> 1–2 cups mixed lettuce
>
> ½ red bell pepper
>
> 1 cucumber
>
> Sea salt and pepper
>
> 1 Tbsp. olive oil
>
> 1 Tbsp. apple cider vinegar

Preparation: Cook the chicken in a preheated pan. Chop the parsley and garlic and rub it on the chicken, once it is cooked. On the side, cut the avocado, red bell pepper, and a cucumber; serve on top of the bed of mixed lettuce. Dress with vinegar, olive oil, sea salt, and pepper to taste.

6. Chicken Lettuce Wraps

Ingredients:

  5 oz. of chicken

  1 Tbsp. low-sodium soy sauce

  ½ red onion, chopped

  5 mushrooms, sliced

  ½ red bell pepper, chopped

  ½ yellow bell pepper, chopped

  ½ orange bell pepper, chopped

  4–5 romaine lettuce leaves

  1 Tbsp. olive or grapeseed oil

  ¼ cup cooking wine

  Sea salt and pepper to taste

Preparation: In a heated skillet, add the chopped onion, bell peppers, and mushrooms; cook for a few minutes. Add the chicken seasoned with sea salt and pepper and continue to cook over medium heat. Once the chicken is golden brown, add the cooking wine and the soy sauce and cook until the liquid is reduced. (Remember to be careful with the amount of soy sauce since it contains a lot of sodium.) Place the lettuce leaves on a plate and serve the chicken on top.

7. Chickpea Salad

Ingredients:

> 1 cup cooked chickpeas
>
> 1 handful of spinach
>
> 1 cup cooked broccoli
>
> 1 medium carrot, grated
>
> ½ avocado
>
> 1 handful of almonds, chopped

Dressing

> 1 Tbsp. olive oil
>
> 3 Tbsp. apple cider vinegar

Preparation: In a bowl add the spinach, broccoli, grated carrot, avocado, and chickpeas (you could use canned, organic, no-sodium chickpeas); mix, and add the almonds and dressing.

8. Mexican Chicken Salad

Ingredients:

> 5 romaine lettuce leaves, chopped
>
> 5 oz. grilled chicken
>
> 1 cup black beans, cooked
>
> 3 Tbsp. guacamole (see page 173)
>
> 2 Tbsp. fresh salsa (see page 154)

Preparation: In a bowl, add the chopped lettuce leaves, mince the chicken and add it to the bowl, add the cooked black beans, top with the guacamole and fresh salsa!

9. Fish Tacos

Ingredients:

> 6 oz. cooked white fish
>
> 4 big leaves of romaine lettuce
>
> 3 Tbsp. guacamole (see page 173)
>
> 3 Tbsp. fresh salsa (see page 154)

Preparation: Grill the fish, seasoned with sea salt and pepper to taste; once cooked, mince it. On each lettuce leaf, add some of the fish and top with guacamole and fresh salsa.

10. Asparagus and Salmon

Ingredients:

> 6 oz. of salmon
>
> 1 handful of asparagus
>
> ½ avocado

Preparation: Preheat oven to 400°, season the salmon with sea salt, pepper, and honey, wrap in aluminum foil, and bake for about 10–15 minutes. Steam the asparagus; once cooked, sauté them on a hot skillet with a little olive oil and season with sea salt and pepper. Place the asparagus on the plate forming a bed and top with the salmon, served with half of an avocado.

11. Turkey Meatballs with Veggies

Ingredients:

      1 lb. ground turkey breast

      1 onion, chopped

      2 garlic cloves, chopped

      1 celery stalk, chopped

      1 red bell pepper, sliced

      1 small head of broccoli

      1 small handful of asparagus

      1 small handful of green beans

      1 Tbsp. coconut oil

      Sea salt and pepper

For the Sauce:

Ingredients:

      1 small onion, chopped

      1 garlic clove, chopped

      2 tomatoes, chopped

      1 bunch of cilantro

      Sea salt and pepper

Preparation: In a bowl mix the ground turkey, onions, garlic, and celery, season with sea salt and pepper. Form into meatballs. In a heated skillet, add the coconut oil and brown the meatballs, set aside. Steam the broccoli, asparagus, and green beans; once cooked, sauté with the red bell pepper. In the same skillet, add the onions; once they look translucent, add the garlic, tomatoes, and cilantro, season with sea salt and pepper, and cook for a few minutes. Add the turkey meatballs, lower the heat and cover to continue the cooking process for about 20 more minutes.

12. Chicken Fajitas

Ingredients:

> 5 oz. chicken breast
>
> 1 small onion, sliced
>
> ½ red bell pepper, sliced
>
> ½ green bell pepper, sliced
>
> Sea salt and pepper

Preparation: Grill the chicken seasoned with sea salt and pepper, and cut into strips. In a heated skillet, add a little bit of olive oil, add the onions and bell peppers, season with sea salt and pepper over medium-low heat. When the veggies are almost ready, add the chicken strips, mix, and cover over low heat for a few minutes.

For the Salad

Ingredients:

> 1 cup mixed lettuce
>
> 1 medium tomato
>
> ½ cup cooked broccoli
>
> 5 mushrooms, sliced
>
> ¼ red onion, sliced
>
> ½ red bell pepper
>
> 2 Tbsp. vinegar
>
> 1 Tbsp. grapeseed oil
>
> Sea salt and pepper

Preparation: In a bowl; add the lettuce, chopped tomato, broccoli, mushrooms, onions, and red bell peppers, season with sea salt and pepper, add the vinegar and the oil; mix well.

13. Grilled Chicken Thai Salad

Ingredients:

> 5 oz. grilled chicken breast
>
> 1 cup mixed lettuce
>
> 1 carrot, grated
>
> 1 medium tomato, cut
>
> ½ red onion, sliced
>
> ¼ cup unsalted peanuts
>
> 1 handful cilantro leaves
>
> A few basil leaves, chopped
>
> ½ avocado
>
> 1 Tbsp. honey
>
> 1 tsp. mustard

Preparation: Grill the chicken with sea salt and pepper. In a bowl, add the lettuce, carrot, onions, tomatoes, cilantro, basil leaves, and the peanuts; mix well. Add the chicken, cut into strips, and top with the avocado. Combine the honey and the mustard, season with sea salt and pepper, and drizzle over the salad.

14. Minestrone Soup

Ingredients:

> 1 cup white beans or 6 oz. of chicken breast
>
> 2 zucchini, chopped
>
> 3 celery stalks, chopped
>
> 4 garlic cloves, minced
>
> 1 onion, chopped
>
> 2 carrots, chopped
>
> 1 bunch of spinach
>
> 2 Tbsp. tomato paste, low-sodium
>
> 10 fresh basil leaves
>
> 1 bunch of parsley
>
> Sea salt and pepper to taste.
>
> 1 Tbsp. olive oil

Preparation: Add water to a pot and cook the presoaked beans; you should be able to squeeze them easily with your fingers when cooked. If you are using chicken, boil the chicken breast and prepare a good basic chicken stock. Add olive oil to a heated pot, cook the onions, add the garlic, celery, carrots, and zucchini, cook for a few minutes and add some water or chicken stock and let it simmer for about 10 minutes. Add the beans or the chicken, lower the heat, and add the tomato paste, basil, and parsley leaves, add sea salt and pepper if needed. Serve hot.

15. Colorful Chicken Salad

Ingredients:

> 3 cups leafy greens
> ½ cup shredded carrot
> ½ cup shredded cucumber
> 1 celery stalk
> 1 chopped tomato
> 2 slices of avocado
> 5 oz. of cooked chicken breast

Dressing:

> 1 Tbsp. olive oil
> 1 Tbsp. white vinegar
> 1 Tbsp. amino sauce (or low-sodium soy sauce)

Preparation: Chop and shred the veggies. Slice the chicken, place it on top of the veggie bed, and add the dressing.

16. Chicken with Sautéed Vegetables

Ingredients:

> 5 oz. of chicken breast, sliced
> 1 onion
> 1 medium tomato
> ½ zucchini
> 5 asparagus
> 1 Tbsp. mustard
> 2 tsp. of amino sauce (or low-sodium soy sauce)
> Sea salt and pepper to taste

Preparation: Cut the vegetables and reserve ½ of the onion for the chicken. In a previously heated pan, add a few drops of grape or coconut oil; sauté ½ the onion with 1 tsp. of amino sauce, until brown. While the onion is cooking, season the chicken with sea salt, pepper, and mustard; remove the onion and cook the chicken. In a different preheated pan, sauté the veggies with 1 tsp. of amino sauce and just a few drops of coconut or grape oil. Place the chicken onto a plate with the onion on top and the veggies on the side.

17. Tuna Salad with Green Beans

Ingredients:

> 1 low-sodium can of tuna, in water
>
> ½ shredded carrot
>
> ½ chopped onion
>
> 1 chopped celery stalk
>
> Sea salt and pepper
>
> 1 Tbsp. olive oil
>
> 1 handful of green beans
>
> 1 garlic clove

Preparation: In a bowl, mix the previously drained tuna, carrot, celery, onion, and sea salt and pepper to taste. Mix well with 1 Tbsp. olive oil. On the side, steam the green beans and then sauté them with a little grape or coconut oil, chopped garlic, sea salt, and pepper to taste.

18. Tuna Salad with Avocado and Mixed Lettuce

Ingredients:

> 3 cups mixed lettuce
>
> 1 carrot, shredded
>
> ½ cucumber, shredded
>
> ½ avocado
>
> ½ cup tuna salad (chopped onion,
> celery, 1 Tbsp. grape oil, sea salt, and pepper)

Dressing:

> 1 Tbsp. rice vinegar
>
> 1 Tbsp. sesame oil
>
> 1 Tbsp. honey
>
> Sea salt and pepper

19. Egg Omelet with Spinach and Arugula Salad

Ingredients:

> 1 whole egg
>
> 3 egg whites
>
> 1 onion, chopped
>
> 1 medium tomato, chopped
>
> 5 mushrooms, sliced
>
> Sea salt and pepper
>
> 3 cups arugula

Preparation: Mix the eggs and veggies and cook in a hot pan. Let it bubble, and flip. Lower heat and cover for a few minutes.

Dressing:

> 1 Tbsp. olive oil
>
> 2 Tbsp. vinegar
>
> Lemon

*Note: Use your creativity and remember to avoid starchy carbo-hydrates at dinner, even if they are whole wheat. You can replace the lettuce for a different green vegetable.

20. Turkey Tacos (protein style)

(Here, we are going to use romaine lettuce, instead of taco shells!)

Ingredients:

> Ground turkey breast, cooked with tomato, garlic, onion, sea salt and pepper.
>
> 3 romaine lettuce leaves
>
> ¼ cup fresh salsa (see page 154)
>
> ½ cup guacamole (see page 173)

Preparation: Once the meat is cooked, divide it into each lettuce leaf, add the fresh salsa and guacamole on top, and enjoy!

21. Ceviche with Asparagus and Avocado

Ingredients:

> 8 asparagus
>
> ½ avocado
>
> 6 oz. of corvina or cod
>
> 3 limes
>
> ½ red onion, chopped
>
> Sea salt to taste
>
> 1 Tbsp. grape oil

Preparation: Cut the fish, squeeze the limes, add sea salt and the onion, mix, cover, and put it in the fridge for 15 minutes. Boil the asparagus in a pan with a little water, once it evaporates, add sea salt, pepper and a little grape oil. Serve the ceviche with avocado and asparagus.

*Note: I hope that you understood that these are just some examples to help guide you. Remember to be creative and play with all the delicious ingredients that you find! Also consider that if you consistently struggle with hunger, your body type and exercise level may require larger portions!

Let's keep up with the healthy lifestyle!

If you really need a hand to have a healthy and happy lifestyle, I recommend you to go to my website, Fat Loss Fiesta. You will find recipes, motivation, exercises and much more.

You can get it at www.FatLossFiesta.com.

Chapter 13

SMART DECISIONS

The simple choices I made saved my habits. They are the ones that kept me going and made it all easier.

However, changing your lifestyle to be healthier and in shape takes time; it's something that you have to be prepared for, constantly. Eating healthy means that you have to cook your own meals, because you need to know exactly what you are eating. This is very difficult at the beginning because you will have a lot of temptations. Those temptations will be so strong that they will take over your willpower and will be hard to ignore.

I don't want to discourage you; I just want to make sure that you know the importance of taking this step. And I want to let you know that a little preparation makes it all the easier.

MAKE TIME TO LOSE WEIGHT

Most people don't have much free time, and for this to work, you need time to prepare your healthy meals.

I chose to do it on Sundays. Every Sunday afternoon, I would cut and separate the lean meats (turkey, chicken breast, and fish) in measured portions, for every day. I would wash and cut the vegetables, cook the brown rice and mix a ton of lettuce and raw vegetables for my salads. I would also get all my snacks in order, such as almonds, apples, walnuts, broccoli, strawberries, etc.

This really worked, because when I felt hungry, my food was ready to eat. This didn't even give me the time to *think* about cheating. The secret is to be 100% prepared when it is time to eat. Have your food and drinks ready for the time when hunger strikes.

Pack your lunch so you are not tempted when you are at work and your coworkers try to convince you to eat out or grab some pizza. When you do the job of preparing your fresh and healthy meals, eating healthy becomes easier. You will get used to the routine and it will become a habit—and that's the whole point!

It may seem like a waste of time to sacrifice a couple hours on a Sunday, but it was vital to reaching my goal. Picking one day a week to prepare will make things easier for you, too!

SLIM DOWN WHEN YOU EAT OUT

You also need to make the best choice possible when you eat out. I don't recommend people eating out during the first 21 days of this new lifestyle, because it can be hard to choose a healthy meal when you are still learning to choose the best options.

However, I know that restaurants are a part of our lives, so use these tips when you eat out.

Order baked, roasted, or grilled chicken. Never ask for fried foods. Order vegetables, a salad, and little olive oil and vinegar on the side (always on the side!). Do not drink alcohol, sodas, or juices. Always get cold water.

Don't be afraid of asking the waiter to modify your meal. The majority of restaurants don't mind, and your requests are normally a quicker choice for the chef.

Oh! And when you first sit down, tell the waiter, "Do not bring the bread, please!" This is a trick restaurants use to increase your insulin levels and make you eat more.

Choose your sides wisely. Many times we choose a healthy main dish, such as a baked, roasted, steamed, or grilled lean meat, but then we ruin it by asking for French fries on the side! We need to be smart when we choose our sides. Many restaurants offer healthy sides such as asparagus, broccoli, or zucchini. Some even offer steamed, mixed veggies. When this is an option, choose it.

For breakfast and lunch, find words such as whole wheat, multi-grain, fiber, rye, barley, quinoa, wild or brown rice, buckwheat, and wheat germ.

Eat like a child. One of the main problems of eating out is that the portions are too big. When this happens, you have many choices. First, see if you can order a smaller size. If there's no alternative, you can order an appetizer from the kids menu! You may think it is silly to order a kid's portion meal, but most of the time, this is what is going to save the extra calories. And always remember that you will be the last to laugh when you look at yourself in the mirror and see an amazing woman looking back at you—all because you chose wisely.

Another option is to find someone to share the meal with. My husband and I do it all the time. If you are ready to order and no one else wants to share, ask the waiter to put half the portion on your plate, and the rest in a to-go box! You will not only avoid overeating, but you will have lunch ready for tomorrow!

If you follow this advice, you will be able to keep a social life, enjoy a night out, and still look good.

It's not so hard, right? Follow these strategies, and you will see a *big* difference!

Chapter 14

BE ACTIVE

Let's be completely honest. There's no need to beat around the bush. Eating healthy helps you lose weight, but to really look good...you have to exercise!

Our bodies were designed to be active and in constant movement; not to be sitting down watching television or at a desk, in front of a computer. We pay the price when we don't activate our body. When we exercise it, it rewards us back. It helps to eliminate toxins, reduce stress, and improve our mood.

This is not something I'm making up to torture you—this is a scientific fact! Exercising helps our body release endorphins. These chemicals interact with our brain receptors and give us a greater sense of happiness.

These sensations have been described as similar to the ones obtained by morphine! The difference is that exercise does not have side effects or create addictions, like the actual drug; it just creates a different way of looking at life and a renovated self-confidence.

The sensation is so incredible, you would think you would have to convince people *not* to do it. However, we always lose track and end up in the same sedentary life as before.

Why does this happen?

Well, most of it is due to the bad information that we read, daily. When we hear the word "exercise," we think about body-builders lifting weights at the gym, or we think about runners running on the treadmill for hours, and we are told that this is how we are supposed to do it. They assure us that if we want to see results, we have to work hard.

The pictures in magazines of people working out look more like a torture routine than something that we can include in our daily lives. That's because, while they were busy filling up their magazines with crazy routines, they forgot that the most important part of reaching goals is having fun in the process!

Exercising should be fun, something that we would *want* to do. It is the time that you take for yourself, and it's a space where you can forget about everything else. The more you enjoy it, the more motivated and easier your workouts will get.

It doesn't matter where you begin. You are not here to compete with Bill Biceps or Rhonda Runner, because if you do, you may fail.

You have to discover what you like to practice. We all have different personalities. We all like different things. But it doesn't matter what we do, as long as we keep our muscles moving, pumping blood, improving each day, and overall, having fun exercising, instead of seeing it as a punishment.

Maybe you like to go out and socialize—you could go to the gym and spend time with your friends. That's fine. Maybe you are a nature lover and love fresh air, and you would rather go for a walk or jog at the park. That is an excellent idea. Maybe you prefer to exercise at home, while you watch your favorite television show. It doesn't matter. Do whatever you wish, but *just do it!* This will give you the best results, in less time.

Personally, it doesn't matter where I am; I need to listen to music. At home, I turn up the volume while I work out, and if I'm at the gym or walking around, I carry my iPod with me. Listening to my favorite songs gives me the extra push to enjoy my workouts, without thinking about it. Time flies and when I notice my watch, I'm already done for the day!

So, focus on what you enjoy. Find the routine that makes you happy; it does not matter what it is. There is no reason to be unhappy when we exercise! You are here to get in shape and be healthy. Nobody is making you, but you are doing it to look and feel good; so enjoy yourself and let endorphins run through your body.

Whatever you do to exercise, it is your business. As I said, the idea is for you to do what makes you happy. You can go out for a walk or a run. You can run on the treadmill or swim in a pool. It doesn't matter what you choose to do, as long as you choose something that you enjoy and that helps you get out of the sedentary lifestyle that you have been living in for years, because it has been inhibiting your weight loss!

It is as simple as starting with a few small changes in your daily life to see great results. For example, take the stairs instead of the elevator. Park your car further away from the door when you go shopping. Walk to nearby places, instead of taking your car; or bike *with* your kids, instead of watching them do it.

If you ask the majority of people, this is not even considered an exercise. What this is about is choosing the healthiest alternative, instead of the easiest. It may not seem to be enough or it might appear to be a waste of time, but trust me; make these small changes in your daily life and you *will* see results.

FIND A WORKOUT PARTNER

Sometimes, starting a new activity can be boring if we do it by ourselves. In my experience, I have found that if you have a training partner, it will be easier to commit to going to the gym. A training partner is someone that can make you responsible, even as *you* are making *them* more responsible.

Even when you don't feel like training, knowing that someone is waiting for you will force you to get out of your comfort zone, even if reluctantly. Of course, once you are there, you will be happy that you have someone to help you through this process. Also, a training partner is healthy and friendly competition.

Maybe some of you don't want to enroll in a gym. The first few months, I recommend that you do go to a gym. It is a place where you can get inspiration to lose weight and be healthy. Also, let's be honest, if you have never trained or haven't trained in years, do you really think you will get motivated at home? It's hard to find the motivation to begin changing your lifestyle when you're at home, surrounded by your normal routine and activities.

On average, a gym membership can cost, per day, what a person would easily otherwise spend on a coffee, a doughnut, or a chocolate bar.

Your health is worth it and I know that you will be glad to have made the investment. You are never going to change anything, if you don't really set out to do it.

Once you have started your gym routine, don't be afraid of mixing up your exercises. Your body will respond better to variety. Go to a spinning class or bring a friend to kick-boxing. Both activities offer a great cardiovascular exercise and help strengthen the muscles.

Right about now, you should be experimenting and seeing changes. You are noticing that, for real results, you have to change out of your bad habits into good ones.

Chapter 15

HOW TO MAKE THIS A LIFETIME TRANSFORMATION

Congratulations for wanting to be healthier and happier! The fact that you are on the last chapter of this book shows me that you are really motivated and ready to make some amazing changes in your life and your body. Since I know you are going to succeed, I want to tell you something else.

Once you start to put everything I have shared with you into action, I can assure you that pounds will start to disappear, and you will feel healthier and look great. You will be an inspiration to others. Many won't believe how good you look, and you will be their motivation to change their lives.

But it doesn't have to end there! Now is when you have to keep your mind and body working together. This first step has set the perfect stage for you to lose weight quickly and easily.

Now you can lose unwanted weight and inches, easier than ever before.

You have taken the first and most important step. The hard job is done. Now it is the time to reward yourself with what you see on the scale, and most importantly, in the mirror. That reward will be waiting for you in FatLossFiesta.com, my fully loaded program that I used to lose 50 pounds in 90 days—and have kept off for the past 5 years!

Fat Loss Fiesta is the next step in your transformation. This system has worked for thousands of people, letting them get amazing results in short amounts of time, and I know that when you go to www.FatLossFiesta.com, you will finally get the body that you have always wanted!

TRANSFORMATION STORIES

I want to make sure that you are convinced that this "New You" transformation story is not only mine, and so, I want to share with you some testimonies from people like you, who were also sad, desperate, and discouraged about their bodies, their health, and their lives, but took the challenge seriously and achieved amazing, drastic changes.

These are some of the success stories that my clients have sent me. Check them out so that you can also get inspired, and see that it is possible to have success, if you follow this plan.

I want to remind you that these are some of my most motivated and disciplined clients. You can obtain amazing results if you follow the food and exercise plan, but, if you don't put in the effort and follow the plan as it was designed, the results may vary. Your discipline level matters! These stories were chosen to inspire you and also to help you understand that you will not get results magically if you don't do the job. I can assure you that if you give yourself the opportunity to change your food and exercise plan, with this program, you will also get amazing results that will stay with you forever.

DAMIRA: FATLOSSFIESTA.COM CLIENT

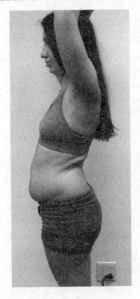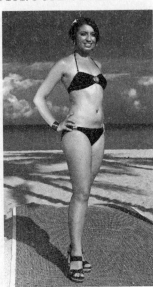

"When I was overweight, I felt bad about myself. Every time I looked at myself in the mirror, I felt depressed and cried. It is hard to explain. I felt fat, ugly, unattractive.... I think it is very hard for us women to feel like that.

"I was always sad and did not want to go out. I felt heavy; I did not want to go shopping, because I felt frustrated with my size. It was a very depressing time. I was not healthy and I felt horrible.

"But now, I feel fabulous. I lost 24 pounds, and now I feel sexy and attractive."

*Results may vary with each individual

OSWALDO: FATLOSSFIESTA.COM CLIENT

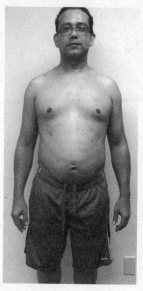 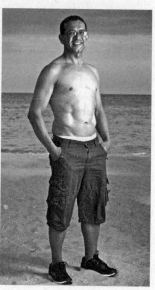

"One day, I took a picture of myself with my phone and when I saw it, I said to myself, This has to stop! I have to do something about this, now! I have to change and take control of my life and health!

"Now, my life is different. I have a new job and I'm starting a new chapter in my life. I see everything in a very positive way, and I was definitely born again.

"I lost 22 pounds, and this is the new Oswaldo. If I could do it, you can do it too."

*Results may vary with each individual

DREE: FATLOSSFIESTA.COM CLIENT

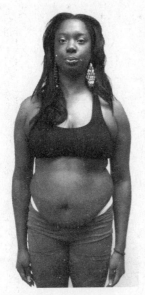 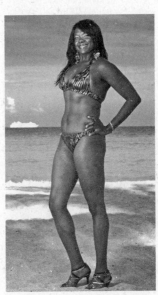

"My name is Dree, I am 34 years old, and I'm from Charleston, SC.

"I have lived in Miami for two years, and even though I like to go to South Beach, I had never been to the actual beach, or even worn a bikini, due to being overweight.

"In January, I decided to change my life and take control of my health. I have lost 25 pounds and if I did it, you can do it too."

*Results may vary with each individual

RENE: FATLOSSFIESTA.COM CLIENT

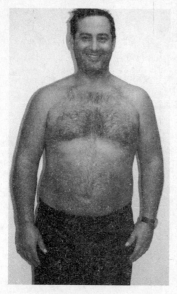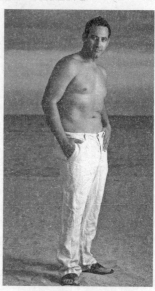

"I went from being a young actor, single at 30, traveling the world, living in Los Angeles and New York and making movies in Hollywood and Broadway shows, to being a proud dad of 4-year-old twins.

"I was always very thin, but back when my twins were born, they were premature and were in the hospital for 2-and-a-half months. This changed my whole life. I focused on saving their lives and didn't notice how it was affecting my personal life; it got to the point where I forgot about me. I gained 40–50 pounds in four years, and this kept me away from my career as an actor.

"I was very happy to be a father, but I was unhappy with myself. Then I told myself that I had to do something to lose weight and take back my career as an actor. Ingrid and her program motivated me to not feel obligated, but to feel excited to make this change in my life, and I did it.

"I lost 40 pounds and I am taking back my career and my life, and I feel great. No one can stop me. You can do it too. The challenge is for you to take back control of your life."

*Results may vary with each individual

THISBY: FATLOSSFIESTA.COM CLIENT

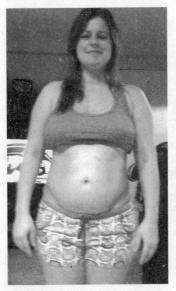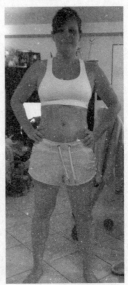

"When I first started the challenge, I had no expectations of success, because nothing had worked for me before this.

"I had just given birth, six months previously, and I thought I would lose the weight, eventually. I didn't exercise, because 'I didn't have time.' Then, one day, I saw a picture of myself published, and it hit me: I realized that if I didn't do anything, I would never lose weight.

"That was the day I decided to give the program a chance. I saw that the food was great and easy to make. I took it, day by day, and before I knew it, 21 days had gone by and the first change was good. I didn't lose much weight, but I had burnt fat. So I kept going, and 90 days later, I had lost 6 sizes. I couldn't believe it!

"Now, I feel beautiful, full of life, strong, and overall, healthy! When I started the program, I did it to find the old Thisby; it turns out, I found a better one!"

*Results may vary with each individual

ANONYMOUS FATLOSSFIESTA.COM CLIENT

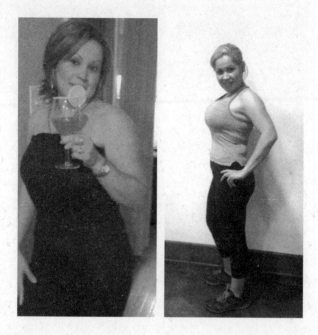

"When I saw my before-and-after pictures, all I could say was 'Thank you Ingrid, for changing my life!' I always talk about you. You are the example of perseverance and you help women all over to regain their confidence."

*Results may vary with each individual

ANONYMOUS FATLOSSFIESTA.COM CLIENT

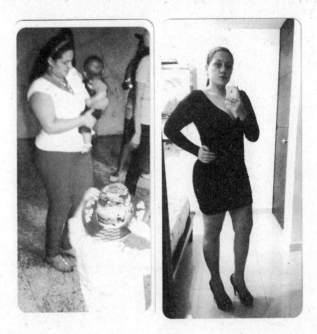

"I thank God for putting you in my way; thank you for teaching me to live a healthy life; thank you for motivating me; and thank you for being my example. Here is my before and after picture. I lost 26 pounds in 3 months and I went from being a size 14 to a size 9. I'm still working on slimming down. I send you my love; you are my teacher, my example, I love you!"

*Results may vary with each individual

ABOUT THE AUTHOR

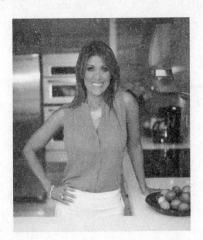

Before inspiring others to change their lives, we must first change our own lives. Ingrid Macher is not afraid of change. Born in Bogotá, Colombia, she came to the United States, searching for the American dream. Now a professional, a wife, and a mother to two girls, she is helping people around the world to improve their quality of life.

After fighting her own weight gain and almost dying in an emergency room at seven months pregnant due to a terrible asthma attack, Ingrid knew she had to take control of her life. She came up with a fun, effective, and practical system to lose weight, and soon lost 50 pounds in 90 days. This system helped her cure her asthma, which lead her to stop taking all kinds of medicines, and it gave her the energy and confidence that she desired. After seeing her clients—busy mothers, overweight adolescents, and even a Hollywood actor—get similar results, Ingrid knew she had discovered something special. So her life mission became to share her knowledge with the most people possible!

As a certified holistic health coach (The Institute of Integrative Nutrition, or IIN) and personal trainer (World Fitness Association), Ingrid is accredited without a doubt. But what makes her a different kind of expert, in health and physical aptitude, is her incredible ability to motivate people to make their dreams come true.

When Ingrid talks, people listen; and lately, she's been talking a lot! She has been featured in El Nuevo Herald, FOX International, MSN, Sirius XM Radio, and dozens of other media channels. She is frequently invited to Telemundo and CNN, where she has been called the "new diet guru who discovered the method that has revolutionized the world of health."

Her articles have received enthusiastic responses and are published weekly in *MamasLatinas.com* and *The Huffington Post*. They can also be found in magazines such as *Miami Shoot Magazine*, *Latina Magazine*, *Gal Time*, and many other digital and print media.

Her YouTube channel has broken records with more than 9 million viewers in its first nine months. More than 500,000 subscribers anxiously wait for the next video. More than 6.8 million Facebook fans show their gratitude for all the advice and motivation they receive about nutrition and physical aptitude, which has helped so many to improve their lifestyle.

After spreading her message to millions of people, many would consider it a mission accomplished. But Ingrid will not stop. She keeps expressing the same motivation that has led her to success, in a short amount of time; the same energy she transmits to her clients, for them to achieve the same incredible results. All of this motivates Ingrid to keep working hard for not only her clients, but all the people who are looking for a healthier and happier life.

YOU CAN FIND HER ON:

Facebook: http://facebook.com/Burn20

Her blog: http://GetHealthyGetHot.com/

Twitter: http://twitter.com/Lose20

Instagram: http://Instagram.com/Lose20

YouTube: http://Youtube.com/GetHealthyGetHot

And on her program, where you will get all the continuing help you need: http://FatLossFiesta.com/